KV-212-859

CONTENTS

ACKNOWLEDGEMENTS

I would like to extend my thanks to all the complementary health associations and institutes which kindly furnished me with career information. Also to Cheryl, who took me on my first step to a healthcare career.

Laurel Alexander

Chapter 1
SO YOU WANT TO BE
A THERAPIST

I qualified as a reflexologist when I was 41, two years after being diagnosed with breast cancer. In fact it was the experience of surviving cancer that acted as a portal into the healing profession. When I left school, I wanted to be a nurse, but with the contrariness of teenagehood, became a window-dresser in a fashion shop instead. So for almost 25 years I ignored my interest in health. As the years went on, I developed a growing interest in mind, body and spirit matters, working more and more in the helping professions, until at 41 I stepped confidently into a new career as a complementary therapist.

Do you know why you want to be a therapist? Can you say what's fuelling your interest and motivation to work in a healing profession? You need to work from the inside out to understand your motivations and to realise where you might fit in if your health career is going to be successful. To find the answers, you should understand what you need from your work, eg autonomy and why you want to do it, for instance, to make a difference. As you become increasingly aware of your work motivations, then you can analyse if you have the aptitude to be a therapist and the discipline to learn new skills. When you've done this groundwork, then you need to go 'outside' and research the marketplace.

I live in Brighton, a town rich in complementary practitioners so there was plenty of encouragement to study for a health career. But how did I choose which complementary therapy to train in? The factors I took into account included: how acceptable the complementary therapy was with the public and orthodox medical profession, how I wanted to work with people, how far I was prepared to travel for training and how long I was prepared to study. My answers? Reflexology ranks as one of the more acceptable therapies with the general public and orthodox medicine.

> **FACT FILE**
>
> A study of the professional organisation of CAM (complementary and alternative medicine) bodies was commissioned by the Department of Health in 1999 (Centre for Complementary Health Studies, Exeter University) and suggested that:
>
> - there are approximately 50,000 CAM practitioners in the UK;
> - there are approximately 10,000 statutory registered health professionals who practise some form of CAM in the UK;
> - up to 5 million patients have consulted a CAM practitioner in the last year.

I wanted a touch therapy, but not one that was too intimate, such as massage. There were three or four opportunities to gain valid reflexology qualifications locally. I chose an intensive course with much study that lasted one year and was accredited by The Association of Reflexologists. Upon qualification and further market research, I decided that although reflexology was valid on its own, to put reflexology with a stress management practice would widen my market – and it has.

You might be a school leaver or graduate looking to step into a health career, or you might be looking for a second (or third) career, or returning to the workplace after a break. You might be seeking to add a different income strand to your portfolio of work (as well as being a health professional, I'm also a writer and trainer). You could be seeking to add another health-related discipline to your existing healthcare skills.

There is increasing interest in complementary therapy in the UK and by choosing a career in this field, you will be opening yourself up to a wealth of opportunity, both on personal and professional levels.

THE DIFFERENCE BETWEEN ALTERNATIVE AND COMPLEMENTARY MEDICINE

The BCMA (British Complementary Medicine Association) has defined alternative and complementary thus:

'Alternative is where the therapist is trained to a level in OM (orthodox medicine) such that he/she can be an alternative to a medical doctor i.e. can make a medical diagnosis (e.g. osteopath or chiropractor) while Complementary means that the level of training in OM does not permit this but is sufficient for the therapist to complement an Alternative therapist or a doctor (with the doctor in clinical control of the case).'

(Excerpt of a transcript submitted to the House of Lords by the chairman of the BCMA, Complementary and Alternative Medicine – Call for Evidence.)

Some call complementary medicine 'alternative', which suggests 'come here instead of there', but it would seem as if the word 'complementary' is best suited to an integrated healthcare system. Complementary medicine doesn't seek to replace orthodox medicine but to work alongside it to provide the best service to the patient or client. There are two ways to define a successful therapist. One is by the number of clients or patients they have – a full appointment book must mean the therapist is good and produces results. The other is the dedication a therapist puts into working in integrated healthcare, for example with the NHS, GPs and other healthcare professionals.

'Complementary and alternative medicine is a broad domain of healing resources that encompasses all health systems, modalities, and practices and their accompanying theories and beliefs, other than those intrinsic to the politically dominant health systems of a particular society or culture in a given historical period.'

(Cochrane Collaboration – an international network of individuals and institutions committed to preparing, maintaining and disseminating systematic reviews of the effects of healthcare.)

TRAINING

There is a need for training at a number of levels in the field of healthcare. Practitioners in CM (complementary medicine) and OM (orthodox medicine) need awareness training in each other's therapies to allow reasoned dialogue and understanding between them. This is in line with

---

FACT FILE

Currently, there aren't many rules and regulations applying to complementary practitioners, but here are some of the general statutory regulations of CAM, from the Department of Health:

- The Food Safety Act 1990 controls the sale and supply of non-medical products for human consumption, which includes some products associated with complementary medicine.
- The provisions of the Trade Descriptions Act 1968 and the Consumer Protection Act 1987 are enforced by local authority Trading Standards Officers, and apply to professions, including complementary therapists, that make claims for the goods or services they sell.
- There is legislation relating to specific illnesses and medical conditions – for example, cancer and venereal disease – which prohibits non-medically qualified individuals from purporting to cure, or in some cases treat, them.
- Some local authorities require the licensing of premises used for activities that include acupuncture, massage and other special treatments.

HRH Prince Charles' action in establishing the Foundation for Integrated Medicine with a mandate to develop a partnership of OM and CM to deal

with the health of the nation. Training in the CM field is moving towards national occupational standards, through Healthwork UK and the Qualifications Curriculum Authority. Similarly CM therapists using OM would be expected to train to the appropriate OM level.

THE FUTURE

More people than ever are seeking to take control of their healing processes, which includes being proactive with the orthodox healthcare professions and working with their technology and advances. However, people are also seeking natural healing through homeopathy, chiropractic and other therapies. Another issue that affects how people choose their healing processes is the caring aspect. When we visit a GP, time is of the essence and we may not always feel we have been listened to. When we visit a complementary therapist, although we pay, we receive time and a holistic sense of healing. By holistic I mean not only are the symptoms treated, but our lifestyle, stress levels, diet and psychological profile are also taken into account. Many GPs argue that they do provide a holistic healing process, but time and financial constraints frequently don't allow this to truly happen.

The future of health is integrated healthcare where orthodox and complementary approaches work together for the benefit of the patient. And you can be part of this major change by becoming a complementary therapist. If you feel inspired to take your new career further, read on about the mainstream therapies you can choose to train in.

Chapter 2
THERAPY OVERVIEW

This chapter provides an overview of 11 complementary therapies: acupuncture, the Alexander Technique, aromatherapy, chiropractic, herbalism, homeopathy, hypnotherapy, massage, nutrition, reflexology and shiatsu.

ACUPUNCTURE

This ancient system of healing was first recorded in China, Japan and other Eastern countries more than 4000 years ago and is based upon detecting disharmonies within a person's body and mind. These are determined by asking questions about presenting symptoms, lifestyle, sleeping patterns and emotions as well as examining the tongue, its colour, shape and coating, and taking a series of pulse readings on both wrists. A traditional diagnosis is then made leading to a treatment plan which will primarily involve the use of very fine needles on acupuncture points (precise locations on pathways of energy called 'meridians'). The needles affect the flow of energy (called 'Chi') through the meridians and thereby stimulate the mental and physical healing energies.

Acupuncture is rooted in the Taoist philosophy of change, growth, balance and harmony. The philosophy outlines the principles of natural law and the movements of life – yin and yang, the Five Elements, the organ system and the meridian network along which acupuncture points are located. The original Taoist records also contain details of pathology and physiology, which provide the theoretical foundation for acupuncture today, some 2000 years later.

There is no government legislation in the UK covering acupuncture at present. This means that anyone, including doctors, physiotherapists, etc can give acupuncture treatment without any training whatsoever.

THE ALEXANDER TECHNIQUE

The Alexander Technique, developed by the Australian actor Frederick Mathias Alexander at the turn of the 20th century, is a way of improving posture and movement, to enable the body to work in a more relaxed and efficient way. Alexander suffered recurrent bouts of hoarseness, which were severe enough to threaten his acting career. He came to suspect that his problems were the result of something he was doing, and set about a journey of self-examination to discover the cause and hopefully cure himself. After several years observing and analysing his reactions, he found that the key lay in the relationship between the head, neck and back. Alexander noticed that when he came to speak, he immediately stiffened his neck and pulled back his head. He developed a series of orders to prevent what he termed his 'pattern of mis-use' that not only cured his vocal problem but also helped his general health and well being.

Alexander had originally thought that these problems were particular to him. However, he began to notice the same patterns in others and, using his own experience, he developed a way of teaching that he called the Alexander Technique. Through gentle manipulation and verbal instruction, Alexander helped pupils to become more aware of the way they used their bodies and to develop greater conscious control of their poise and movement. As well as teaching individuals Alexander set up a three-year training course to teach teachers how to use the Technique.

Alexander Technique professionals consider themselves not as healthcare professionals treating patients, but as teachers teaching students. Typically a course of treatment or instruction lasts around 30 half-hour sessions, during which the student is made aware of the way he or she holds and moves their body. Many students report greater energy and physical mobility, and the Alexander Technique is especially popular with actors and musicians.

AROMATHERAPY

Essential oils were used in ancient Egypt and many came from China and India where there is evidence they were in use for a thousand years before the pharaohs. The scientific study of the therapeutic properties of essential oils was started in the 1920s by Rene-Maurice Gattefoss, a French cosmetic chemist. One day he burnt his arm and plunged it into the nearest cold liquid, which happened to be lavender. He noted the pain lessened and that his wound healed quickly and left no scar. From then on, he dedicated his life to researching essential oils and coined the term 'aromatherapy'.

Essential oils are made from plants and trees, specifically the stems, fruits, roots, petals, bark, leaves, seed and resin. There are around 400 essential oils in general use today, with research confirming that they are anti-viral, anti-bacterial and anti-fungal. Essential oils possess distinctive therapeutic properties, which can be utilised to improve health and prevent disease. Their physiological and psychological effects combine well to promote positive health.

After diagnosis to determine which oils would be most appropriate, highly concentrated essential oils are mixed with a carrier oil and massaged into the skin. These natural plant oils are applied in a variety of ways including massage, compresses, baths and inhalations.

CHIROPRACTIC

Chiropractic originated over 100 years ago in the US. It is a health profession concerned with the diagnosis, treatment and prevention of mechanical disorders of the musculoskeletal system and the effects of these disorders on the function of the nervous system and general health. After diagnosis, which involves the use of X-rays, assessment of medical history and a physical examination of muscles and joints, treatment consists of a wide range of specific manual techniques designed to improve the function of joints and relieve pain or muscle spasm. Chiropractors use their hands to adjust the spine and joints where signs of restriction in movement are found, improving mobility and relieving pain. This treatment is known as 'manipulation' or 'adjustment'.

McTimoney Chiropractic

This is a unique branch of the chiropractic profession in the UK. It is named after its originator John McTimoney who developed his whole-body style of treatment in the 1950s, from those techniques originally taught at the first college of chiropractic, The Palmer College. It is a particularly gentle, whole-body variation on this manipulative technique. It aims to correct the alignment of the bones of the spine and joints of the body, to restore nerve function, to alleviate pain and to promote natural health. McTimoney chiropractors check and subtly adjust the bones of the skull, thorax, spine, pelvis and limbs, relieving problems throughout the entire structure.

HERBALISM

Surviving Egyptian papyri dating back to around 1700 BC record that many common herbs, such as juniper and garlic, have been used medicinally for around 4000 years. Other cultures with a history of herbal medicine include the ancient Greeks and Romans, the Chinese (as long ago as 2500 BC a Chinese herbal listed 365 remedies) and the Indians. The philosophy behind Western herbalism has been strongly influenced by Ayuvedic medicine (the traditional systems of medicine in India). In Britain, the use of herbs developed along with the establishment of monasteries. In Wales and Scotland, Druids and other Celtic healers are thought to have an oral tradition of herbalism where medicine was mixed with ritual and religion. As scientifically inspired medicine rose in popularity, herbal medicine went into decline, although it was still practised in rural areas. The National Association (later Institute) of Medical Herbalists was formed in 1864 to maintain standards of practice and organise training. Gradually public interest in herbal medicine has increased, especially over the past 30 years. Today, globally, herbal medicine is three to four times more commonly practised than conventional medicine.

Herbal medicine draws on the whole of the plant world for its sources, including trees, shrubs and seaweed plus other plant materials such as berries, bark and flowers. They can be taken in capsules, fluid extracts, decoctions, infused oils (external use), compresses, poultices, suppositories or teas.

Chinese Herbal Medicine (CHM)

CHM is an ancient system of healthcare that has undergone continual development over the centuries as the causes of illness that afflict mankind have evolved. In China it is not an alternative form of therapy, but is used in the state hospitals alongside modern medicine. CHM is a complete medical system that is capable of treating disease in all its forms. Although a practitioner will treat the complaint, the traditional view places great importance on preventing disease before it occurs.

HOMEOPATHY

This therapy has been established for about 200 years and is an effective and scientific system of healing that assists the natural tendency of the body to heal itself. It is founded on the belief that all symptoms of ill health are expressions of disharmony or imbalance within the whole person and that it is the patient who needs treatment, not the disease.

In 1796 a German doctor, Samuel Hahnemann, discovered a different approach to the cure of the sick, which he called homeopathy (from the Greek words meaning 'similar suffering'). Like Hippocrates 2000 years earlier he realised that there were two ways of treating ill health: the way of opposites and the way of similars. Take, for example, a case of insomnia. The way of opposites (conventional medicine or allopathy), is to treat this by giving a drug to bring on an artificial sleep. This frequently involves the use of large or regular doses of drugs that can sometimes cause side effects or addiction. The way of similars, the homeopathic way, is to give the patient a minute dose of a substance such as coffee, which in large doses causes sleeplessness in a healthy person. Perhaps surprisingly this will enable the patient to sleep naturally.

The aim of homeopathy is to stimulate the body's own healing ability and recover the balance that has been lost. Minute doses of the homeopathic remedy are diluted in water and re-diluted several times, a process known as potentisation, which paradoxically is believed to increase its potency. Homeopaths take special account of the mental and emotional state of the patient.

HYPNOTHERAPY

Healing through the hypnotic state can be traced back as far as the Druids, who referred to the altered state as 'magic sleep'. However, it was not until the mid-19th century that the current methods of capturing a patient's total concentration through eye contact and verbal suggestion were established, and in 1955 the British Medical Association approved hypnosis as a valuable technique in the world of healing.

Hypnotherapy uses the power of the mind to help heal physical as well as emotional problems. It helps the patient discover the underlying emotional and psychological causes of their ailments. A hypnotherapist will attempt to find out as much about the client and their problem as possible during the first visit, to try to establish the relevant psychological factors and the appropriate mode of treatment. In hypnotherapy you will be relaxed and, by talking in a firm but monotonous voice, the therapist will put you into a hypnotic state – neither asleep nor awake. The therapist will then try to extract information from your subconscious mind in order to find the cause of your problem, possibly by taking you back to your childhood for your earliest memories. Suggestions may be made to your subconscious which will be related to your problem. At the end of the session you will be brought out of the hypnotic state feeling calm, relaxed and re-energised.

MASSAGE

As far back as 3000 BC, massage was used as a therapy in the Far East. Hippocrates recommended that a massage using oils should be taken daily after a perfumed bath so as to maintain health. The word 'massage' is most likely to have come from the Greek word 'Massein', meaning 'to knead', or the Arabic word 'mas'h', meaning 'to press softly'. Massage grew in popularity in the 19th century when Per Henrik Ling, a Swedish fencing master, created the basis for what we now know as Swedish massage. This therapy works on the soft tissues of the body and its relaxing effects help both muscles and joints. During the 1970s, *The Massage Book* was published by George Downing, which introduced the concept that the state of a person would be assessed by a therapist in a holistic way and not purely on a physical basis. From this, therapeutic massage was developed to relax, stimulate and invigorate.

A relaxation massage is primarily a de-stressor and doesn't necessarily work deep into the tissue. Remedial massage is aimed at specific muscular problems such as a bad back or a local injury. Sports massage offers a regular MOT for sports people and works deep into the muscles. The whole person is treated using four basic techniques: effleurage (stroking), friction (pressure), percussion (drumming) and petrissage (kneading). Massage is now incorporated into other therapies such as rolfing (tissue massage), aromatherapy, Indian head massage, reflexology and shiatsu.

NUTRITION

A nutritionist is someone who examines our dietary intake and lifestyle so as to discover any imbalances. Food provides us with the energy and vital nutrients necessary to remain healthy and help us should we become ill. We may have an allergic reaction or a food intolerance, which leads to an eruption on the skin. Stomach cramps, vomiting or diarrhoea may occur after eating certain foods. Knowing which foods are responsible is the first step to ascertaining how to go about addressing the problem. Often the only way is to carry out an elimination diet, by excluding certain substances. An initial consultation with a professional nutritionist takes about an hour and a half, during which time diagnostic tests on hair samples, gut permeability and allergies may also be carried out. Once the nutritionist is in possession of all the necessary information, a time-bound programme focusing on which foods to eliminate and which to increase, plus supplements, is incorporated into the person's life.

Naturopathy

Naturopathy is a 19th century word meaning 'nature cure'. Naturopathy aims to encourage health by both stimulating and supporting the body's inherent power to regain or maintain well being. The discipline is based on four principles:

1) that the individual is unique;
2) that it is more important to establish the cause of the condition than to treat the symptoms;
3) that individuals have the power to heal themselves; and
4) that there is a need to treat the whole person and not just the part of the body affected.

It is the use of external and internal remedies that work within the individual and evoke the healing power of the body, for example good nutrition is an internal remedy. Externally, various massage techniques, aromatherapy and herbal liniment make up the naturopathic treatment. Physical, environmental, mental, emotional and circumstantial factors are taken into account. Diagnostic tools such as iridology, where ailments can be traced through the markings, pigmentation and structure of the eye's iris, may be used, or Chinese Traditional Medicine may be applied. Traditional Chinese Medicine (TCM) is a safe and proven healing system. Sessions typically last for 40 minutes. A typical treatment may include acupuncture, massage and corrective exercises. Herbal remedies, dietary advice and various exercises may also be prescribed.

REFLEXOLOGY

Although there is scriptural evidence to suggest that reflexology was being practised as far back as ancient Egypt, Dr William Fitzgerald (an American ear, nose and throat surgeon) founded the science of reflexology used today. He noticed that pressure on specific areas of the body produced an anaesthetising effect on a related area. Developing his theory, he divided the body into ten equal zones that ended in the feet and hands. In the 1930s a massage therapist called Eunice Ingham refined Dr Fitzgerald's zones and developed what is now known as reflexology. She observed that congestion or tension in any part of the foot mirrored congestion or tension in a related part of the body. Therefore, treating the areas of the feet could have a relaxing and healing effect on different organs and tissues inside the body.

Nerve endings, embedded in the feet and hands, travel to the spinal cord and to various parts of the body. Stimulating these nerve endings helps promote relaxation, improve circulation, stimulate vital organs and encourage the body's natural healing processes. Unlike conventional medicine, reflexology works on the underlying problems within the body and works through the body's nervous system.

SHIATSU

Shiatsu literally translated means 'finger pressure'. Chinese Taoist monks were the first to observe our self-healing instincts over 5000 years ago and eventually they formalised these observations into a system for treatment. Their theories involved acupuncture, moxibustion (which involves the stimulation of energy through the use of a burning herb either on a needle or over a specific accupunture point) and herbology. Chinese medicine was introduced to Japan by the Chinese Buddhist monks about 1000 years ago, and by adding acupuncture points to their already existing massage techniques, shiatsu emerged in Japan and is now a fully accepted medical treatment, authorised by the Japanese Ministry of Health and Welfare.

Shiatsu is based on the same principles as acupuncture but without the needles, concentrating on meridians or energy lines. The idea, as in acupuncture, is to balance the life energy in the body that is disturbed when we become ill. Through a series of finger pressures all over the body along the meridians or pathways, shiatsu can rebalance the body's energies, regulate the function of the organs and improve circulation. By releasing the body's natural energy flow, our self-healing process is able to take place. Shiatsu practitioners often use their elbows, knees and feet as well as their fingers during therapy, but they seldom use the palms of their hands, unlike other traditional Western contact therapies.

Several therapies have been left out of this chapter because the training for them is too vague or because the therapies themselves lack enough credible research. But you might like to explore them for yourself. They include: flower essences (eg, Bach Flowers), Reiki, spiritual healing, kinesiology, polarity therapy, hydrotherapy, colour therapy, rolfing and iridology.

Now that you have some idea of what the mainstream complementary therapies are, discover if you've got the basics of what it takes to be a good therapist.

Chapter 3
HAVE YOU GOT WHAT IT TAKES?

Most people working as a healthcare professional are people-oriented and have a caring nature, which needs to be expressed in a proactive way. Because complementary health has more of a holistic reputation and application, complementary therapists need to be able to balance being 'touchy-feely' with a good business sense. Many complementary therapists have good people skills, are able to work holistically and know their therapy inside out – but, as most therapists are self-employed, all this is pointless if you can't market yourself, your skills and your therapy.

For the purpose of this chapter, I have assumed the occupational skills and knowledge needed for each therapy (training for these is covered in Chapter 4). What is maybe more important is to highlight the skills, knowledge and personal qualities any complementary therapist needs in order to run an efficient and useful practice.

SPECIALIST KNOWLEDGE

Knowledge of the law in relation to health. There are laws affecting how any health practitioner may work. The UK and the rest of Europe have specific laws regarding orthodox and complementary practitioners. You need to be fully aware of these. It is crucial that you keep yourself up to date with health and safety (H&S) information and practice. This is obviously related to insurance but, more crucially, to the well being of your clients. There are H&S issues relating to the use of equipment, oils, tinctures and other preparations; to your treatment room, to clients moving on and off couches or other equipment; to clients moving into and out of and within premises. Don't forget also the H&S issues relating to yourself such as working with infections and working with members of the public in your home.

These contacts will provide you with further information on health, law and H&S:

- David Evans, Health Care Lawyer. Advice on health law matters such as consent, negligence, clinical risk management, dispute resolution, confidentiality, etc. Several health law links. Tel: 020 8286 1445. Website: www.davidevans-law.co.uk
- Health & Safety Executive. Website: www.open.gov.uk/hse/hsehome.htm. For information about legal H&S requirements.
- Herbal medicine has strict regulations and if you want to research these further, contact the professional bodies for herbalism given in the appendix of this book.
- It is against the law to say you can cure certain diseases, for example cancer. It is also against the law to set up in certain medical professions without the appropriate qualifications, for example dentistry. These kinds of laws should be made clear to you during your health-related training.

General knowledge of other therapies. OK. So you're an expert in your therapy. Great. But your clients may be having other therapies and you need to know a little about them so that you can balance your treatment. It may be, for example, that you as a reflexologist are working with a client helping to relieve their stress-related symptoms, but it might also be useful if your client were to see a homeopath or herbalist for additional health support. You need to know the benefits of other therapies and how one therapy could complement (or work against) another.

Basic understanding of psychology. Whatever type of complementary practitioner you are, you need to have a basic understanding of the human psyche. We're not talking psychotherapy here or obtaining a degree in psychology, but it is useful to have a working knowledge of what makes people tick, for three reasons. First, psychology is helpful for developing your interpersonal skills. Secondly, a good therapist always needs to understand where they are coming from as well as where a client is. Thirdly, in order to provide a holistic service to clients, you need to be able to read between the lines of what they say (or don't say). They don't always say what they mean – they don't always know what they mean. Being able to understand a client's anxieties about health problems can be helpful to the healing process in general. Another more esoteric reason is to understand how the psychological make-up of a person can affect their predisposition to illness – not only their coping mechanisms but also in terms of how particular characteristics may produce certain physical symptoms or tendencies. A good basic text is *Hilgard's Introduction to Psychology* (Harcourt Brace).

Knowledge of local/national support groups. Working with a client in a healing capacity means not only delivering and supporting the therapy and healing process, it may also mean gleaning an awareness of other problems a client may have that could be affecting their health, such as financial issues. So it is useful to have a resource of referrals to local and national information and support groups.

Interest in holistic forms of healing. Being a complementary therapist means that you don't only treat symptoms, you also take into account personality, lifestyle and other issues relating to the 'wholeness' of a person. An understanding of how the mind, body and spirit interact with each other and how these elements relate to health is therefore essential.

PEOPLE SKILLS AND STRENGTHS

- *Listening skills.* A good therapist knows how to listen properly to others. Listening skills involve not only hearing the words and the tone people use but also observing body language. Real listening means making someone feel that what they have to say is worthwhile.
- *Telephone skills.* You need to be able to handle sales enquiries by phone, and provide reassurance and guidance to existing clients over the phone. You are likely to be liaising with other health professionals and support services, so you need to be able to handle negotiation processes over the phone.
- *Questioning skills.* Clients may vaguely state their health problem and it's up to you to use questioning techniques to elicit the right information from them.
- *Helping skills.* In addition to a basic knowledge of psychology, it can also be of benefit to have some helping or counselling skills to draw out more information from the client.

- *Networking skills.* The best way of getting work and developing your practice is to network. Get yourself out and about: build up contacts and bridges of opportunity.
- *Being approachable.* A practitioner needs to be approachable, not only to get clients but also to encourage clients to talk as part of their healing process.
- *Adaptability.* Adaptability is important because of the speed of change in the marketplace. As you develop your complementary health career, you will find you need to adapt to survive.
- *Physical and mental fitness.* For several complementary therapies, eg, chiropratic or massage, you neeed physical strength. For all therapies you need emotional and psychological fitness as the work can at times be very draining.
- *Reliability.* If you can't make an appointment, you must let the client know. You are responsible for setting boudaries and professional behaviour. That isn't to say, sadly, that your clients will have the same reliability!
- *Giving constructive feedback.* Clients want reassurance that the treatment is working, that they are getting better. The sandwich technique is a good way of giving feedback: you offer a positive opener, then tactfully deliver the feedback and close with a positive ending.
- *Ability to facilitate change in others.* Often a client's lifestyle adversely affects their emotional, psychological and physical well being. At times like this, you may need to make suggestions to the client for positive change (which they may accept or ignore).
- *Minimising anxiety in your clients.* You need to be able to recognise anxiety in others and be able to reassure them both over the treatment procedure and their healing process.
- *Promoting other people's self-esteem.* When health problems strike, a person's self-esteem can take quite a knock, and it is important for you to help them boost their confidence as part of the healing process.
- *Trustworthiness.* This has a lot to do with being able to keep a confidence and offering unconditional support. Clients need to be able to trust you, not only with their health problem and their body, but also with their anxieties and worries.
- *Being positive.* You must always be realistic but positive. There is a difference between a cure and healing. A cure is when a positive change can happen in the body or mind. Sometimes a cure is not

possible, but healing is. Healing, in this sense, comes more from helping the client to accept their condition and building self-esteem.

- *Calmness.* As a therapist, you will run the gamut of experience, some of it not always pleasant, but however much you might want to scream, save it until the client has been treated and has gone.
- *Objectivity.* While it is important to have empathy and sympathy with clients, it is also important (for professional ethics and you own well being) to be objective.

BUSINESS SKILLS

- *Marketing skills.* Whether you want to work for yourself or be employed by someone else, you need to be able to market yourself. Marketing includes advertising, getting yourself on referral lists from GPs and other therapists, writing articles and books on your therapy, participating in exhibitions, giving talks or workshops. If you want to work for yourself, you need to consider public relations too.
- *Interview/meeting skills.* An interview is where you come under the limelight, where you need to specifically sell yourself. In a meeting you may still need to sell yourself, but there is more of a sense of negotiation. You may need to have initial meetings with clients prior to agreeing to work together, there are team meetings in clinics or you may need to meet with other health professionals. If you want to teach your therapy for adult, further or higher education you will need to attend an interview.
- *Time management skills.* All practitioners need to manage treatment time, as well as balance daily, weekly and monthly tasks such as dealing with finance or marketing.
- *Numeracy and literacy.* These skills might seem obvious, but in order to write up your treatment records, a good command of English is helpful. You might want to write reports or articles (a good way of building your reputation) and don't forget your promotional material.
- *Organisational skills.* If you are going to work from home or run your own business, you need to be organised. Time management, administration skills and problem solving are important, and you also need critical thinking skills – and a sense of ruthlessness in order to

dump what you don't need and focus on what you do need.

■ *Referral skills.* You need to be able to recognise your limitations and know when a client needs something you cannot provide. Then you need to know who might be able to fulfil the client's need.

■ *Teaching skills.* Sometimes as part of delivering a health-related service, you will find yourself teaching clients certain techniques or exercises they could do to help the treatment be more effective. You might also teach a course or workshop related to your therapy; this is an excellent way of extending your skills, making money, spreading the word and possibly getting new clients.

■ *Problem solving skills.* How do you modify your treatments to suit your clients? How do you market your business? How can you get more clients? What do you do with difficult clients? How do you find the money to invest in that new treatment couch? Effective problem solving and decision making skills will make these issues easier to address.

At this stage it's important that you have the personal qualities to be a complementary therapist. It's your driving spirit, motivation and positive attitude that will form the foundation for a successful career in health. Gaining the knowledge and learning the skills come after that – in the next chapter in fact.

Chapter 4
TRAINING ROUTES

Currently it is legal for anyone in the UK to practise complementary therapy without having had any relevant training (except in the cases of osteopathy and chiropractic; these are protected by statute). Many would-be therapists have jumped on what seems to be an easy bandwagon without qualifications. But you will be caught out, either through malpractice or because you don't know enough, don't produce results and won't get the clients.

However, it isn't always easy to spot the genuine qualifications because of the huge number of pseudo-qualifications. There are many colleges offering 'massage courses by distance learning' or 'learn hypnotherapy via our cassettes and workbook'. Many places of learning offer certificates and diplomas that encourage you to think you are studying for a recognised qualification – but you aren't. The way to spot the genuine qualifications is to ask who accredits the certificate, diploma or training. By this I mean, who is the validating body eg, City & Guilds, The National Council for Psychotherapists, RSA, The Association of Reflexologists. Some places of learning have their own 'accreditation'. If the course is being offered by a further education college, university or established school/college of medicine, you can check their validation by going to the lead body. But if the piece of paper is offered by a college or school that says it's 'internally validated' – be wary.

When I decided to train in stress management, I spent hours surfing the Web to find a genuine qualification. There were several stress management certificates and diplomas, but when I delved deeper I discovered that there was no accrediting body. The pieces of paper meant nothing. The stress management course I finally settled on was a distance learning course taken over 10 months with a specific college that has this particular course accredited with a lead body. Then I checked out the lead body – which was genuine.

> **FACT FILE**
>
> Some of the therapies traditionally considered to be complementary
> are being taken up by doctors. Some medical schools are now offering
> complementary medicine familiarisation courses to undergraduate
> medical students, while others offer modules specifically on
> complementary medicine.

You might be tempted not to get qualified. But you won't be taken
seriously by the orthodox health profession or by clients if you can't
prove that you have taken an accredited and genuine qualification course.
See the appendices for a list of education providers and lead and
professional bodies.

CURRENT STATUS OF TRAINING

Acupuncture – The British Acupuncture Council is the largest group
representing acupuncturists in the UK and has been involved in the
formation of an Independent Accreditation Board for Educational
Standards. This was established to ensure that no college or course would
be advocated by the Council without being scrutinised by an
independent board.

The Alexander Technique – There are approximately three Alexander
Technique associations. Each of these groups uses a formal accreditation
process to screen membership but does not require members to have
graduated from a recognised college. The educational requirement for
membership ranges from three years full-time to four years part-time
training.

Aromatherapy – The Aromatherapy Organisations Council represents
the 'majority of professionally qualified aromatherapists' who work in
the field of complementary medicine, through its 12 professional
member associations. The therapists recognised by the Council have
trained to standards defined in that body's core curriculum. The
Aromatherapy Organisations Council's minimum educational
requirement for membership is nine months part-time, which adds up to
180 hours, plus 50 supervised treatment hours.

Chiropractic – This is one of two CAMs with professional bodies
established by statute (the other is osteopathy), and has clear guidelines
on education set by its regulatory council (the General Chiropractic
Council, GCC). The GCC has the advantage that by law all those
practitioners calling themselves chiropractors must abide by the training
standards set by the respective regulatory bodies. Practitioners of
mainstream osteopathy, chiropractic, acupuncture, medical homeopathy
and herbal medicine now recognise their limits of competence and will
refer patients whose problems do not lie within those limits, for
conventional medical treatment.

Herbalism – The European Herbal Practitioners Association (EHPA)
was established in 1993 to unify the herbal medicine profession. It has
been working towards bringing herbal practitioners from a variety of
different backgrounds under one body with a common core curriculum.
Their core curriculum lays down basic standards of training and is
'science based', in that it teaches the basics of conventional medicine and
points out the limits of competence of trained herbalists. To reflect the
growing number of BSc degree programmes available in this subject, the
core curriculum is aimed at a four-year university course. Educational
requirements for membership in the herbal medicine organisations range
from four years of full-time study to two years of part-time study.

Homeopathy – The largest homeopathic professional organisation, the
Society of Homeopaths, is working to develop national occupational
standards in homeopathy with the assistance of Healthwork UK. The
Society says, 'There has been quite a development in education … things
have evolved in the last 22 years quite dramatically; during that time we
have seen the introduction of full-time courses equivalent to
undergraduate degree training. We now have two university degrees, BSc
(Hons) degrees in homeopathic education. The interesting thing about
these degrees is that the conventional medical part of the education, which
contains basic anatomy, physiology, pathology, research methodology etc,
is part of the curriculum which has been written by doctors'.

Hypnotherapy – The UK Confederation of Hypnotherapy Organisations
(UKCHO) is the first umbrella body to represent 30 organisations that
have come together to enhance the professional status of hypnotherapy
and to provide a united voice on matters such as training standards,

occupational standards, ethics and legislation. UKCHO also represents the profession of hypnotherapy to government agencies and the general public. It can supply a list of training bodies and accrediting organisations (Tel: 0870 6070422).

Massage – There are nine organisations representing massage therapists, but many massage therapists may also be members of aromatherapy organisations as the two therapies are often practised together. The proportion of massage therapists in organisations that use a formal accreditation process to screen membership is small, but all require members to graduate from a recognised college and almost all require continuing professional education. For membership the time committed to educational requirements ranges from 100 hours to 1600 hours.

Nutritional Therapy – The Nutritional Therapy Council (established in 1999) is an umbrella body for nutritional therapists, which focuses particularly on educational standards and on developing national occupational standards for the profession. The largest nutritional therapy organisation is the British Association of Nutritional Therapists. It believes that the Nutritional Therapy Council will be able to co-ordinate training colleges. Currently educational requirements for membership of the different nutritional therapy bodies range from four years full-time to two years part-time. All bodies require members to graduate from a recognised college, and over half use the formal accreditation process to screen membership.

Reflexology – There are approximately ten bodies representing reflexologists. Most practitioners are in organisations that use a formal accreditation process to screen membership, all requiring members to graduate from a recognised college. Educational requirements for membership range from 60 to 100 hours of training. Recently all the identified reflexology organisations have agreed to work together within a new reflexology forum, launched in September 2000, with the aim of identifying new national occupational standards for the discipline.

Shiatsu – There are approximately five organisations representing Shiatsu practitioners in the UK. All the identified organisations use a formal accreditation process and require members to graduate from a recognised college. The educational requirement for membership varies between 150 and 500 hours of training.

FACT FILE

Continuing professional development (CPD) is vital if CAM professionals are to keep up with new developments in their field; it is also a mechanism that can be used to encourage research, understanding and inter-professional collaboration.

HOW DO YOU LEARN?

Training for complementary therapies is usually undertaken in a classroom situation. You may attend a course on a daily (full-time), weekly or monthly basis. Some courses are held over occasional whole weekends. Some are provided via distance learning with support by email, post and the phone. Beware of any courses where you learn by workbook, audio or video tape alone with no support at all.

FUNDING YOUR TRAINING

Individual Learning Account (ILA)

ILAs are a way of helping you pay for your learning. Backed by the government and supported by learning providers, trade unions and employers, ILAs offer a package of discounts that make it easier for you to get into learning. If you are aged 19 or over you can open an Individual Learning Account. You can claim a £150 contribution if you're one of the first million account holders to book learning and put up £25 of your own money, or you can claim a 20 per cent discount up to the value of £100 per year towards a wide range of learning, including some activities which could be classed as recreational and do not necessarily lead to qualifications. There are some specific exclusions for the £150 payment and the 20 per cent discount. You could also choose to take advantage of the 80 per cent discount (to the value of £200 per year) on what you pay towards some types of learning – these are limited to a range of computer literacy and introductory maths courses. Most lead to recognised qualifications such as City and Guilds Awards, GCSEs and key skills 2 maths, but you do not have to achieve qualifications in order to benefit from the 80 per cent discount. Once you've applied successfully for an ILA, you will receive an Account Card. You will then be able to use this with any of thousands of participating learning providers.

FACT FILE

To open an ILA account and claim the discounts call 0800 072 5678 or visit the
      ILA Web site www.my-ila.com/.

Access Funds

Money from Access Funds is allocated to students who have serious financial difficulties or who might not otherwise have access to higher education. Some colleges and universities have their own separate hardship funds. Either way they decide who is eligible – and for how much. Ask the college or university for more details.

Career Development Loans

If you're planning to do some learning related to a job and you can't afford to pay for it, a Career Development Loan (CDL) may be the answer. You can apply to borrow between £300 and £8000 to pay for:

■ up to 80 per cent of your course fees, as well as
■ the full cost of books, materials, and
■ other expenses such as travel and childcare, and
■ living expenses if it's a full-time course.

You don't need to pay back the loan until you've finished studying and you're in a job. The scheme is operated by the Department for Education and Employment in partnership with four high street banks (Barclays, Clydesdale, The Co-operative and The Royal Bank of Scotland). The loans are to pay for up to two years of training (or up to three years if the course includes work experience). The Department pays the interest on the loan for the period of the training and for up to one month after it has finished. You then repay the bank over an agreed period at a fixed rate of interest. It may be useful to contact the CDL banks before you apply for a loan to find out how much you would repay in total.

Charities and trust funds

Some educational trust funds and charities will help towards fees, books or equipment. Call at your local library to find contact details, or check with your local college, careers service or education authority to find out whether any organisations near you operate the Inspire, Funderfinder or Moneysearch databases. They match your personal profile to the most likely charities or trusts, saving you the chore of scanning through directories. EGAS, the Educational Grants Advisory Service, may also help you track down funding.

Employers

Your employer may be happy to fund your learning, especially if it relates to your work. Check whether your organisation has a personal development scheme or training programme, or whether they'll allow you paid time off for studying. Larger organisations may also offer sponsorship.

Help for people out of work

If you're unemployed, improving your qualifications can help you find a job. Ask at your local Jobcentre about the New Deal and training schemes. Check whether starting learning will affect your benefits.

Small Firms' Training Loans

Small Firms' Training Loans (SFTLs) are operated in partnership with eight high street banks. The aim is to help businesses employing up to 50 people to pay for work-related education or training. Firms can apply for loans of between £500 and £125,000 to cover training costs, and up to £5000 to cover consultancy advice on training. For information about which interest rates apply to your curcumstances you should contact the participating banks. The banks may offer different terms and conditions and may offer either fixed or variable rates of interest. The minimum repayment period is one year and the maximum seven years. You will normally start to make monthly repayments within a month of the end of the deferment period.

Student loans

There are no longer grants available to students in higher education to pay for living costs. Instead, you need to apply for a student loan. Your local education authority will tell you the level of loan you are entitled to. Loans are repaid once you've finished your course and are earning an income. Go to www.dfee.gov.uk/loan 2000/index.htm for more information.

Further financial help

There may be extra help for certain students or students on certain courses. For instance, there are supplementary grants for:

- disabled students, students with dependants, single-parent students, students with travel costs and those who've recently left care;
- part-time students – help with fees, loans for course-related costs, Disabled Students Allowance and Access Fund help;
- NHMs bursaries – available for some healthcare courses;
- those on benefit – you may be eligible for housing and council tax benefit;
- teacher training courses – some teaching courses attract particular types of additional funding.

In the Appendix you will find a selection of the wide variety of training and courses on offer. You can apply directly to further education colleges and universities for courses on complementary therapies as well as the lead bodies (which will have their own accredited learning centres). You can also search the Internet for training in complementary therapies.

You've decided on your complementary therapy. You've got yourself on the way to a qualification. Now how do you find work?

FACT FILE

Further contacts:

- Career Development Loans (CDLs) – 0800 585 505 or branches of Barclays, Co-operative, Clydesdale or The Royal Bank of Scotland
- Educational Grants Advisory Service (EGAS) – 0207 249 6636 (9:30am to 1pm)
- Financial Support in Higher Education – 0800 731 9133
- Student Loans Company – 0800 405 010
- The learndirect helpline – free – 0800 100 900 or www.learndirect.co.uk
- Your local education authority, public reference library, careers office, college library or Jobcentre.

Chapter 5
WORKING FOR YOURSELF

When you have qualified as a complementary therapist, you will, in essence, be working for yourself, at home and in a variety of other settings. Many therapists are 'portfolio workers' – they have more than one strand of income. You might choose to work part-time for an employer to ensure some kind of steady income while you build up your complementary health practice, where you most likely will be self-employed.

If you have never been self-employed, you might find the idea a bit daunting. Some benefits include:

- improving your self-confidence;
- working the hours you want;
- working at something you enjoy;
- the potential to make unlimited money;
- learning about business.

MARKET RESEARCH

Before you embark on working for yourself, you need to do some market research. In fact, even when you're up and running, you still need to have your finger on the public pulse.

Knowing current trends is vital to building a healthy business – trends not only in your professional field, but also in terms of market fluctuation. For example, who are the types of people who will pay for your therapy? Is your therapy based on need eg bad backs, or curiosity? If your locality is flooded out with your type of therapy are you willing to travel further afield for work? Is there a trend towards teaching self-help or selling products within your therapy? What are the market gaps? Can you create a niche for yourself, for example baby massage?

QUESTIONS FOR MARKET RESEARCH

- What are the personal factors affecting the purchasers of your service or product – their interests, income, age, marital status, social class, family size, sex?
- What are the purchaser's reasons for buying the service or product?
- What is the size of your potential market?
- Is your potential market likely to grow in the future?
- How do the potential customers/clients buy – Yellow Pages, mail order, etc?
- Who are your competitors (strengths and weaknesses, product or service, prices)? How do they market their service or product?

BUSINESS SKILLS

Having qualified as a therapist and knowing you have a needy market waiting to give you their money is half the battle. The other half is using your business skills so that you can run and develop your business successfully.

RAISING CAPITAL

You could start up a complementary health business with your own money. However, you may need premises and expensive equipment. Sources of financial help include:

- banks
- private loans
- money from local authorities
- government initiatives
- overdraft facilities
- leasing or hire purchase
- turning personal assets into cash.

BUSINESS SKILLS ASSESSMENT

Rate yourself on the following:

market analysis	YES	NO	SOME
drawing up business plans	YES	NO	SOME
setting prices	YES	NO	SOME
advertising	YES	NO	SOME
public relations	YES	NO	SOME
selling	YES	NO	SOME
keeping accounts books	YES	NO	SOME
installing a system of credit control	YES	NO	SOME
negotiating credit terms	YES	NO	SOME
drawing up cash flows	YES	NO	SOME
drawing up budgets	YES	NO	SOME
product distribution	YES	NO	SOME
stock control	YES	NO	SOME
recruiting staff	YES	NO	SOME

If you really want to build a thriving practice, you need to focus on developing your skills and knowledge across the board of business skills.

Funding for the small business

Grants and funding for new or very small businesses are limited and depend very much on the geographical area in which you run your business.

- If you are unemployed you could qualify for a grant of up to £1380 towards set-up costs.
- Some areas operate the New Entrepreneurs Challenge Fund, which provides a grant of £1000, loans, on-going business support and training.
- You may qualify for a grant to meet 50 per cent of the costs of diagnostic and consultancy support – this could be useful if you plan to develop your business. You will probably have to show 12 months' trading accounts to qualify.
- Discretionary grants may be available under Regional Selective Assistance if you live in or are relocating to an Assisted Area, are creating employment or safeguarding existing jobs. This includes your own job.

> **FACT FILE**
>
> Ask your local Business Links for information about grants and funding for which you may be eligible (Tel: 0345 567765).

- If you live in or are located in the East or West Midlands, you may also qualify for a Regional Enterprise Grant.
- If you live in a rural area you may be eligible for a grant towards the conversion costs of redundant buildings. In 1995/96, almost £12m was contributed to workspace programmes.

The Small Business Service

The UK government recently announced proposals for a new Small Business Service, starting in April 2001.

'A new Small Business Service was also announced. This will have a strong remit to deliver the advice and support that firms need to grow and bring together different parts of the DTI, Better Regulation Unit and the DfEE from April 2001. Modelled partly on the Small Business Administration in the USA, the new service will provide small business with:

- options to cut compliance burden;
- automated payroll service for small employers;
- expansion of quarterly employers PAYE scheme from a limit of £600 a month to £1000 a month;
- new Inland Revenue business support teams to discuss problems with any business within 48 hours;
- new business advice service from Customs and Excise for exporters and importers;
- new Enterprise Support Initiative, including a dedicated helpline for new employers;
- discounts for internet-filed electronic tax returns.

There will also be measures to encourage investment. The Government will extend 40% first year capital allowances for another year, together with proposals for R&D tax credits for small and medium-sized companies.'

(Working Brief, Unemployment Unit & Youthaid Research, Information, Campaigning, 322 St John Street, London EC1V 4NU)

COSTINGS

As part of your costing, you may need to consider:

telephone	furniture	vehicles
computers	premises	your salary
printing	production	other salaries
advertising	clothing	treatment products
publication subscriptions	professional membership	additional training

MARKETING

Mercenary though it may sound when considering a healthcare practice, the only way you are going to get customers and sales is through marketing. Ways of getting your message across to the public include:

posters	ads
sales letters	letterbox drops
press releases	direct mail
radio	TV
public speaking	leaflets
brochures	seminars
forums	sponsorships
agents	writing articles/books

THE LAW AND YOU

Knowing the law and its relevance to your business gives security and credibility. This includes:

- getting professional advice from an accountant;
- choosing a legal form of business identity for your business, ie whether you will operate as a sole trader, a partnership or a limited company;
- complying with business or company name regulations;
- registering for VAT;
- notifying the Inland Revenue and the DSS of your business status;

Safety Issues

When you work from home, you are in a vulnerable position, especially if you are a woman.

It is crucial you take all precautions necessary to safeguard yourself and your privacy. The Suzy Lamplugh Trust is the national charity for personal safety. It aims to create a safer society and enable people to live safer lives, providing practical personal safety advice for everyone. Contact the trust directly on 020 8876 0305.

- considering your need for patents, copyright or trademark registration;
- complying with the laws affecting business premises and trading, including business rates;
- considering the need for a licence eg some towns require you to have a licence in order to practise as a therapist;
- knowing your rights as an employer;
- checking your insurance needs eg professional indemnity.

HOMEWORKING

Many complementary therapists work from home, either entirely or as one of a number of locations. You work the hours you choose, there are no travelling costs, you can create the ambience you want in your clinic and there are no office politics to get sucked into. To help you get the most out of working from home, here are some key tips:

- Lay down ground rules with family and friends so they appreciate the nature of homeworking. Some people think that if you work from home you're not really working. You will need to arrange separate domestic and working space.
- Keep up other interests. It is harder when working from home to leave work problems behind at the end of the working day.
- Try to establish a network of other therapists working from home, to combat feelings of loneliness and to offer each other support for problems.

WEB SITES

Here are some sites that might help you set up in business:

Advertising Standards Authority
www.asa.org.uk/
The ASA aims to promote the highest standards in advertising.

DO$H bookkeeping
www.dosh.co.uk

DO$H Cashbook assumes no bookkeeping knowledge but provides help through on-screen steps and a comprehensive manual. The software allows users to produce a complete record of all receipts and payments, a cash flow summary, a VAT account and bank reconciliation statements for any period, and prints out reports on A4 paper.

Inland Revenue
www.inlandrevenue.gov.uk/home.htm
This site offers questions and answers for the self-employed.

Business Names Register
www.bnr.plc.uk
For a small fee, the Business Names Register will search over 3 million business names and 600,000 registered trademarks to ensure your name does not conflict with anyone else's.

Data protection
www.dataprotection.gov.uk/guide.htm
A 40-page guide issued by the Data Protection Registrar gives advice on how the Data Protection Act 1984 affects homeworkers. As almost all businesses that keep records on clients need to be registered, it is important that you comply. This has been made a lot easier with the assisted pre-filling of forms available on the Registration Line (01625 545740). Copies of the booklet or more information about the Act are available from the Information Line (01625 545745).

Health & Safety Executive
www.open.gov.uk/hse/hsehome.htm
Here you will find information about legal health and safety requirements, many of which apply to small businesses.

Mail Order Protection Scheme
www.mops.org.uk
MOPS acts as a guarantor for advertisers. It protects consumers
buying by mail order if an advertiser covered by the scheme goes bust.
MOPS only covers cash-off-the-page advertising in national daily
newspapers.

Natwest Small Business Planner
www.natwest.co.uk/frontpage/dhtml/index.htm
To download the free planner software, select from the top drop-down
menu 'small business' then follow the links to 'starting a business' then
'setting up a business'.

Planning permission
www.homeworking.co.uk/library/planper.htm
Find out about planning permission and using your home for work.

Trading Standards
www.tradingstandards.gov.uk/
This is your one-stop shop for consumer protection information in the
UK. The site is supported and maintained by ITSA, the Institute of
Trading Standards Administration.

Viking Direct Ltd
www.vikingdirect.com
You can find a vast range of items for offices, shops and warehouses
through this site. Ask for 'the cheapest price' as prices vary between
catalogues.

Yahoo! Small Business
http://smallbusiness.yahoo.com
Tips and advice for building your clientele can be found through this
portal.

Home Business Alliance
www.homebusiness.org.uk/
The HBA is able to offer you a constant supply of valuable, time-saving
and quality information that will help you achieve your business aims.
You'll be plugged into a network of experienced advisers including
accountants, marketing and business consultants, financial experts,

ex-bank managers, educationalists, publishers, authors, tradesmen and craft workers.

You're qualified and have set yourself up in business. You're ready and raring to go. Now where do you find the work? Where are the clients?

Chapter 6
CAREER PATHS

This is the hardest part. As a practising complementary therapist, you need to be constantly looking for work. Even when you have a full diary, you need to be networking and building contacts for the future. You also need the skills for lateral thinking. Clients will not be queuing up outside your door – you will need to go out there, find them and convince them you are the best person for their needs. Research skills are also useful as you need to find out who does what, where, why, and how you might fit in.

Here is a range of opportunities where you might find outlets for your therapy.

THE NHS

There are many collaborative ventures within the NHS, such as the Marylebone Health Centre, a London NHS practice where complementary therapists and GPs work together. You could do some research to find out what collaborative ventures there are in your area. Travelling out of your area occasionally is a good idea – not only for the change of scenery but also to widen out opportunities. One county can have very different attitudes to another.

GPs

GPs are becoming increasingly inclined to provide integrated healthcare to NHS patients, which includes access to CAM.

You could approach practice managers to work in surgeries. Some GPs are more open to this suggestion than others. You need to ensure there is a working space for you and arrange a regular time for you to be there. Also be

Breast Cancer and Complementary Therapies

Brighton has an excellent breastcare unit and as a survivor of breast cancer and a reflexologist, I was given permission to put up a poster for my therapy. Clients phone me and I work on a concessionary basis with them either at my home or theirs.

The unit also has an aromatherapist who comes in one afternoon a week to give one-off treatments to clients.

Integrated Healthcare: A guide to good practice

This book is based on the entries to the 1999 Good Practice in Integrated Healthcare Awards. It includes guidelines for setting up integrated healthcare projects, case studies of the shortlisted projects and sources of further information. Written by Hazel Russo, copies are available from the Foundation of Integrated Medicine (www.fimed.org) at £7.99 plus £1.25 p&p.

clear as to how appointments are going to be made, for example via your phone number, and whether you will do it or the receptionist will do it for you.

Another way of working with a surgery is to put a poster or leaflets in the waiting area (with the permission of the GP and the practice manager) and let prospective clients phone you. Be aware of safety issues if seeing clients in their home).

The NHS Confederation says it supports moves towards integration and that 'This is a process that is already happening and the boundaries of what is considered "conventional" and "complementary" are constantly shifting' (acupuncture in pain clinics, for example).

New Primary Care Guide to Complementary Medicine

Recent surveys have shown that at least 1 in 3 people will use complementary or alternative therapies at some time during their life. Every year more than 1 in 10 will visit a complementary therapist for one of six named therapies: acupuncture, osteopathy,

Methods of Delivery within the NHS

PATIENT

GENERAL PRACTITIONER

(or other member of primary care team) may provide CAM treatment themselves if trained; or refer to:

A member of an on-site multi-disciplinary team (as in the Marylebone Health Centre)

A specialist CAM centre within an NHS Acute Trust (e.g. London Homeopathic Hospital)

A specialist CAM centre contracted by the District Health Authority (e.g. Centre for Complementary Health Studies in Southampton)

An individual, off-site, CAM practitioner contracted by the Primary Care Group or Primary Care Trust

A secondary care service within the NHS Acute Trust that uses CAM (as in some physiotherapy and orthopaedic clinics)

If patient is terminally ill refer to a palliative care unit which provides CAM

Take advantage of District Health Authority Initiatives that may be piloting CAM projects.

(Taken from the CAM Report by the House of Lords, 2000)

chiropractic, herbal medicine, hypnotherapy or homeopathy. GP practices and primary care increasingly provide their patients with access to therapies such as these. A new information pack *Complementary Medicine: Information Pack for Primary Care Groups* was launched during a special exhibition at the House of Commons sponsored by the All-Party Group for Complementary Medicine. It has been produced by the Department of Health in collaboration with the NHS Alliance, the National Association of Primary Care and the Foundation of Integrated Medicine. A booklet designed for clinicians will be provided to every GP practice. A more detailed pack will be sent to all Primary Care Groups and Trusts. Both are designed to inform clinicians and managers, and provide a resource for making sensible and locally sensitive decisions about commissioning the six complementary therapies that are most often provided in the NHS. The documents are also available on-line (www.doh.gov.wh). They provide information on six individual therapies including details of relevant qualifications and the bodies responsible for the registration of medically-qualified and non-medical practitioners. For each therapy information is given on what conditions would benefit most from treatment. No longer regarded as the province of charlatans and the deluded, there is an increasing interest in complementary therapies from politicians and health service managers as well as clinicians. (www.internethealthlibrary.com, July 2000)

BMAS Leads on Integration of Acupuncture into NHS

The British Medical Acupuncture Society (BMAS) welcomes the publication of the British Medical Association's (BMA) report into acupuncture. The BMA's report concludes that acupuncture works, is safe (safer than many drugs prescribed daily by doctors) and should be made available on the NHS. This represents a sea change in the opinion of the medical establishment. The BMAS has been working for many years to integrate acupuncture into the NHS and trains doctors in acupuncture. It is impressive that nearly half the GPs in the BMA's survey wanted to receive training in acupuncture. The BMAS is committed to train more doctors in acupuncture and to integrate acupuncture further into the NHS. The fact that nearly half of the GPs in the BMA survey have arranged acupuncture for their patients and that 79 per cent want to see acupuncture available on the NHS demonstrates that acupuncture has now well and truly arrived in this country. (The British Medical Acupuncture Society, June 2000 www.internethealthlibrary.com)

THE PRIVATE SECTOR

CAM is primarily practised in the private sector with clients directly approaching and paying an independent complementary therapist.

Self-referral to a specialist centre

An example here would be someone who felt they needed pain control and went to a pain clinic which, as well as the orthodox treatments, might offer acupuncture or stress management.

GP referral

Clients will come from the GP to an independent complementary practitioner or specialist centre, whether paid for directly by the client or through health insurance.

Community health initiatives

The Department of Health is keen to emphasise that CAM practitioners are also welcome to play a role in supporting community health initiatives such as their Healthy Workplace Initiative, the Healthy Living Centres and Healthy Schools projects.

Private rest homes/convalescence homes

Not all therapies are suitable for these places. Reflexology, massage and aromatherapy are good bets. Write a letter outlining what you are offering, for example 30-minute reflexology sessions for £10 or a 15-minute Indian head massage for £5. Enclose a leaflet providing your background and qualifications. Maybe you could offer an initial talk to residents and staff or a free session to a staff member. You could visit

---

Chicken and egg

Sonia is 50 and works as a part-time administrator for the NHS. She took a Diploma in Person-Centred Counselling at a local further education college when she was 48. She is building up her hours towards accreditation with the British Association of Counselling (BAC) via voluntary work with a youth aid agency offering individual and group counselling to 18–25-year olds who have referred themselves. One of the biggest problems Sonia has found is that in order to become employed as a counsellor, she needs to be accredited by the BAC. 'It's a chicken and egg situation,' she says. 'If you want to be employed as a counsellor, you need to be an accredited member of BAC. In order to be accredited, you need a certain amount of hours under your belt, but it's hard to get the hours under your belt because you're not an accredited counsellor. So the best way I found to gain the hours is through voluntary sector who aren't quite so demanding.'

---

each home once a month and make sure you have enough clients to make it worth your while – half a day's worth or hopefully a full day's worth.

Natural health clinics

There are clinics in virtually every town, offering a wide range of therapies. Rooms are rented out on an hourly basis, maybe something like £10 an hour or £50 for a half day. Some places allow you to pay as you go, especially when you're starting up; others want you to sign on the dotted line for six months. The advantages of working from a clinic are that there is a sense of belonging, there will be a receptionist to welcome clients and take bookings, the room is cleaned for you and there might be a cross-referral of clients, for instance someone who visits the shiatsu therapist may also want acupuncture.

At the time of writing this book, The Body Shop had a policy of renting rooms in their shops to therapists.

Shared practices

Slightly different to natural health clinics is the shared practice. This is where two or three therapists get together and rent somewhere. They are the resident therapists.

> **The group practice**
>
> Jackie is in her late 30s and after several years of personal development through her own counselling, recently qualified as a counsellor at a local further education college. Prior to and throughout her training she worked full-time shifts for the police as a call operator – and still does. Jackie is now setting up a practice in her spare time with two other counsellors who qualified on the same course. They are renting a room in a business centre and intend to each practice for seven hours per week. They want to run self-help groups in specialist areas such as eating disorders and are going to sublet the room at other times to therapists. All three counsellors went on an enterprise scheme to learn business skills. Jackie would eventually like to go part-time in her job and work the rest of the time in the counselling practice. 'My main issue at the moment is financial. I can't leave my job because the pay is so good because of the shift hours. My husband isn't happy in his job either and would like to change. We're thinking of buying a house as well. So really, both of us need to stay where we are at the moment until we can sort out some basic financial issues. I'm working really hard at two jobs and I am very tired but I feel I'm working towards what I really want to do. All I need is patience – and perseverance!'

OTHER IDEAS

Other ways to ply your trade include:

- Social services in daycare centres offering reflexology.
- Cruise ships in their health and beauty salons offering reflexology, massage, aromatherapy, nutrition or shiatsu.
- High street beauty salons offering reflexology, hypnotherapy, massage, aromatherapy or nutrition.
- Gyms and health clubs offering reflexology, massage, aromatherapy or nutrition.
- Working overseas for charities offering homeopathy.
- Working with special groups, for example children/adults, the elderly

and the terminally ill and offering reflexology, massage or aromatherapy.

■ In the workplace offering reflexology, hypnotherapy, nutrition or massage.

■ Selling related products, for instance:
 – reflexologists could sell health and beauty products for the feet;
 – nutritionsts could sell dietary supplements;
 – herbalists could grow and prepare their own herbal remedies, selling them to clients, retail outlets or other therapists;
 – hypnotherapists could sell videos and tapes;
 – aromatherapists could make their own perfumes and create beauty products. They could package and market a travel care kit or a basic care kit for the home medicine cabinet. They could design their own range of essential oils and massage techniques for sports people and dancers. They could make fragrant products for the home such as air fresheners, bacteria busters, candles, soaps, pot pouris, perfumed pillows and paper. They could make scented gifts for special occasions such as Christmas, birthdays or Valentine's day.

■ Teaching. You could teach your subject on adult education leisure courses or you could teach on a qualification course via a further education college, university or a professional training school. Any therapy or related area could be taught on a leisure basis. Here are some ideas:
 – homeopathy: first aid in the home or homeopathy for children;
 – hypnotherapy: relaxation techniques to overcome fear, or using self-hypnosis techniques to boost confidence;
 – herbalism: natural remedies in the kitchen or using herbs for beauty;
 – massage: massage for babies or for couples;
 – nutrition: better eating for life or the medical kitchen;
 – reflexology: using body reflexology for improved health;
 – aromatherapy: using oils in beauty preparations, or scented gifts.

Here are some further general business ideas for any therapist:

■ writing articles and books;
■ renting room space to other therapists;
■ getting together with one or two other therapists and offering healthy/educational breaks;

- masseurs could offer on-site massage and shoulder massages for the business market;
- nutritionists could set up a weight control clinic

Selling health-related products over the Web

The number of people with Internet access is currently growing at the phenomenal rate of 10 per cent every month, with the value of financial transactions on the Internet doubling every three months. If you have complementary health products that could sell well by mail order, e-commerce might be a useful and profitable outlet for you (I bought my treatment couch through the Internet). People buy online 24 hours a day, seven days a week, 52 weeks of the year. Imagine having access to all those clients!

Setting up a school

Julia is in her late 40s and entered complementary health from the retail industry after recovering from a serious health problem several years ago. She gained qualifications in reflexology, massage and aromatherapy over a period of time before considering starting her own reflexology school (reflexologists can't teach reflexology until five years after qualification). Two years ago, she sought accreditation with the Association of Reflexologists, took the Certificate in Education (a key qualification for teaching adults) with a local college and eventually began successfully recruiting students onto her practitioner certificate course which she runs from the local natural health centre. 'Although the course is recruiting well,' she says, 'I am a relatively inexperienced teacher, which is providing me with a challenge. Now, because of internal difficulties in teaching where I am, I'm thinking of teaching the course from home. I'm discovering that one of the most useful things I can do for my school is PR and marketing. Every so often, for example, I take a few of my old reflexology students into the local shopping mall for an all-day event giving free reflexology treatments to the public. That promotes reflexology as well as my practitioner course.'

In order to sell online, you need to own some Web space where your shop Web site will live and be seen by visitors. Then you need some shop-building software. A good shop-building package will automatically create the correct secure environment for handling credit card orders. You can also receive orders via email and sort out the details and the payment using more traditional means such as getting back to the customer by phone or by ordinary mail. But what do you put on your website? I would suggest you include: company/therapist profile, products and services, prices including delivery if appropriate, some kind of interactive section, eg, quiz, free advice, how customers can contact you, a customer feedback section and other information such as links to associated sites.

THERAPIES AND SPECIFIC CAREER PATHS

Here is an insight into salaries and career paths for specific therapies.

Acupuncture

Salaries vary enormously, anything from £10,000 to £50,000. Acupuncturists work from their private practice, in the NHS and complementary health centres. Some may work in projects such as drug and alcohol services. Many work in GPs' surgeries and others in pain-management clinics.

The Alexander Technique

Teachers are almost always self-employed. Most teachers around the country charge at least £20 for a 30–40 minute session. London fees are higher than in other parts of the country; the average is £25–£35. When fees are paid by a school, the NHS or some other organisation, they will sometimes be lower than those charged in private practice. Most work in private practice with some having additional part-time roles such as working in the NHS in hospital pain-management clinics or in a support centre for cancer patients. Some work in private clinics; others work in the chain of recently launched Boots Wellbeing Clinics. Some work in music and drama academies, some in schools with children and teenagers.

Some go in-house to large companies and provide the Technique to employees (the company provides the room and the session is paid for by employees). Some Alexander Teachers hire a room at a health club.

Aromatherapy

Aromatherapists, depending on their location, charge between £25 and £40 for a treatment. Many therapists look for work in clinics or set up their own practice. Therapists also work on a voluntary basis in old people's homes, hospices, etc in order to gain a wider experience of treating people. Some therapists are medically trained as nurses or physiotherapists and practise aromatherapy alongside their work. There are also those who work within GP practices.

Chiropractic

There is currently a shortage of chiropractors in the UK. As a relatively young profession here, chiropractic also offers exciting research opportunities. There are core fees for treatment ranging from £25 to £50 with extra fees for x-rays. Chiropractors usually work alone or in a practice with other chiropractors.

Mail order herbs

Robert started his healing career in acupunture in his 20s, learnt about orthobionomy (a muscle release technique developed by Dr Arthur Lincoln Pauls), discovered iridology and then took a degree in naturopathy. He is now in his mid-40s and describes himself as a naturopathic herbalist. After several years of being a practitioner of acupuncture and iridology, practising from home and in a London clinic, he started up a herbal business from a back room in his home and now has a thriving mail order and Internet business with premises and employees, selling herbal remedies throughout the world. 'I changed from treating people face-to-face to dealing with people via mail order primarily because of my interest in business and health as opposed to people and health,' he says, 'I wanted to make money, provide a back-end service to practitioners and use my business skills.'

Herbalism

Most herbalists go into private practice working from home, or in a multidisciplinary complementary medicine clinic or GP surgery. A few are employed by the NHS, Boots or some other form of business. Other areas herbalists go into are teaching at the various colleges for herbal medicine (this usually requires some teaching experience or qualification), growing herbs or manufacturing herbal medicines, retail (eg, herbal dispensaries or health shops) and research.

Income is variable, from £100 per week to businesses worth in excess of £1 million. Many herbalists work part time to suit family needs, some have another job either to supplement their income or regard herbalism more as an interest; others work full time and do very well. The higher earners tend to be involved in retail and manufacturing or are very active in promoting themselves as practitioners.

Homeopathy

Professional homeopaths work in homeopathic clinics, above pharmacies, in health clubs, on their own and in clinics with other

---

Third world business

Cheryl is in her late 40s and is a practising homeopath with over 15 years' experience. Her initial interest in natural health arose from a history of back problems and an involvement with osteopathy. An additional interest in nutrition led to her working for Weleda (makers of aromatherapy and beauty products) and through this she developed an awareness of herbalism and homeopathy. As she wanted a career that was flexible enough to go hand in hand with motherhood, she decided to take a part-time course at the College of Homeopathy and began working from home in the early 1980s with help from the Government Enterprise Scheme. Initially Cheryl rented a room in a clinic one day a week. Now she works primarily from home in a dedicated room. She is also paid by a charity to take her skills to third world countries and teaches two days a month in a school of homeopathy. 'A typical working week,' she says, 'covers four consulting days, seeing no more than ten patients per day, plus one day a week for administration. An hour every day is put aside to deal with telephone enquiries. Any time between is filled with study and sending out repeat prescriptions.'

---

alternative/complementary therapists. A small but growing number have begun to work in GP surgeries, although most are in private practice. Fees are from £40–£70 for new patients and £35–£40 for follow-up sessions.

Hypnotherapy

A hypnotherapist may see a client between four and six times, charging in the region of £35–£55 per session. Hypnotherapists are based in their private practice but may run pain relief clinics at hospitals or anti-smoking treatments for large companies.

Massage

Indian head massage fees are between £15 and £25 for a 30-minute session, while a 60-minute massage could bring in £25–£45. Remedial massage fees are around £20–£30 for 30 minutes. You could work from a clinic, health club, salon, hospital, surgery or gym. Many massage therapists work via GP or osteopath recommendation. There could be openings in the developing area of using massage for cancer patients suffering from the after-effects of treatment.

Moving on

Michelle, 33, originally trained as a classical dancer before becoming a fitness instructor in her 20s. She then moved into working with injuries. She now works as a personal trainer and massage therapist offering Indian head massage (having qualified with a local private training school), relaxation massage, remedial massage and sports massage as well as individual personal training programmes. She rents a room in a natural health clinic and another in a local gym, each for one day a week. Michelle also works from a multi-practice health clinic several miles away once a week and does home visits (clients coming via word of mouth) in between. She has recently qualified as an NVQ assessor and is considering assessing fitness instructors. 'I've worked for several years in the field of massage and have always made sure to go on courses to refresh and stimulate me. I think therapists need to reinvent themselves in order to keep their interest alive – and their service tiptop. Now, although I still want to offer treatments, I would like to move into teaching massage and fitness as well.'

Nutrition

Nutritionalists' fees may be between £30 and £70 per hour depending on the location. Many health clubs as well as some private doctors' surgeries employ a nutritionalist. Some nutritionalists write for magazines and papers, some work for supplement companies or health food shops. Some teach and lecture in colleges, others work with sports teams. Other areas of business include support groups such as ADHD (Attention Deficit Hyperactivity Disorder), asthma or AIDS. The majority of nutritionalists work in multidisciplinary clinics.

Reflexology

Opportunities for reflexologists are opening up at a rapid rate, and whilst the traditional route of self-employment is still the norm for most reflexologists, more and more are finding part- and full-time employment. Many reflexologists are now employed by the NHS and businesses are increasingly using reflexology to help cope with the effects of stress; reflexologists are appearing in hospices, care homes, hospitals, clinics, public companies, small businesses, gyms and on luxury liners. Private medical establishments are increasingly offering reflexology as an optional therapy. Some private medical insurance companies are willing to fund reflexology treatment under their policies and many nurses, healthcare workers and midwives are adding reflexology to their repertoire of skills. Doctors who manage their own budgets find that by employing a reflexologist they can save substantially on their drugs bill. Most reflexologists working privately charge their clients between £15 and £30 for a treatment that may last for 45 minutes to an hour. Some reflexologists go on to teach either at FE colleges or in private education.

Shiatsu

Charges for Shiatsu are broadly within the band of £20–£40 per hour, though some practitioners may charge less if in a subsidised or charitable situation; others may charge more. Private practice is the most common mode of working, although shiatsu is being offered in a number of charitable projects such as drug rehabilitation and cancer. A growing area of interest is in the NHS and with GPs, though funding for such activities is currently difficult, as there is no government support or help through insurance schemes.

The appendices offer a range of information on education providers, lead and professional bodies, and further resources. These contacts and the links you make from them should help you step into your new career as a complementary therapist. Good luck.

EDUCATION PROVIDERS

These are a selection of education providers offering learning opportunities in complementary therapies in general, and in specific therapies. Check with each one for validity, mode and cost of learning. The list is by no means exhaustive and there are many excellent providers that have not been included here due to a lack of space.

COMPLEMENTARY THERAPIES

Blackpool and the Flyde College
(Holistic Therapies: Body Massage, Aromatherapy and Reflexology Diploma. Also complementary therapies HND)
Address: Ashfield Road, Bispham, Blackpool, Lancashire FY2 0HB
Tel: 01253 352352

Bradford College
(Complementary Therapies Bsc (Hons))
Address: School of Science & Technology, Great Horton Road, Bradford, West Yorkshire BD7 1AY
Tel: 01274 753333

City College Manchester
(Complementary Therapies National BTEC Diploma)
Address: Wythenshawe Park Centre, Moor Road, Wythenshawe, Manchester M23 9BQ
Tel: 0161 957 1790

Derby University
(Complementary Therapies and Holistic Medicine BA (Hons))
Address: School of Health and Community Studies, Kedleston Road, Derby DE22 1GB
Tel: 01332 621 317

Exeter University
(Complementary Health Studies: Postgraduate Certificates, Diplomas and MA degrees. Also research degrees: MPhil and PhD)
Address: Centre for Complementary Health Studies, Amory Building, Rennes Drive, Exeter EX4 4RJ

Tel: 01392 264 498
Fax: 01392 433 828
Email: CHS@exeter.ac.uk
Website: www.ex.ac.uk

Greenwich University
(Complementary Therapies BSc
(Hons))
Contact: Denise Tiran
Address: Wellington Street,
Woolwich, London SE18 6PF
Tel: 020 8331 8000 or Freephone
0800 005006

Harrogate College
(Complementary Therapies
Diploma)
Address: Hornbeam Park,
Harrogate, NorthYorkshire
HG2 8QT
Tel: 01423 879466

Llandudno College (Health and
Complementary Therapies HND
and Health and Complementary
Therapies HNC)
Address: Llandudno Road,
Rhos-on-Sea, Colwyn Bay,
Conwy LL28 4HZ
Tel: 01492 546666

North Tyneside College (Body
Massage, Aromatherapy, Indian
Head Massage
Certificate/Diploma)
Address: Embleton Avenue,
Wallsend, Tyne and Wear
NE28 9NJ
Tel: 0191 229 5000

Pembrokeshire College
(Complementary Therapies –
National Diploma BTEC)
Address: Merlins Bridge,
Haverfordwest, Pembrokeshire
SA61 1SZ
Tel: 01437 765247

Perth College (Complementary
Therapies HNC)
Address: Crieff Road, Perth,
Perthshire and Kinross
PH1 2NX
Tel: 01738 632020

Tower Hamlets College
(Complementary Therapies –
NVQ Level 3)
Address: Poplar Centre,
Poplar High Street, Tower
Hamlets, London E14 0AF
Tel: 020 7538 5888

Wales University
(Complementary Therapies Level
2 Module – 40 CATS Points)
Address: The School of Health
Science, Singleton Park, Swansea
SA2 8PP
Tel: 01792 518531

Westminster University (BSc
(Hons) in Acupuncture,
Chiropractic, Complementary
Therapies, Herbal Medicine,
Homeopathy, Nutritional Therapy
and Therapeutic Massage)
Contact: Campus Admissions
and Marketing Office

Address: Centre for Community
Care and Primary Health,
115 New Cavendish Street,
London W1M 8JS
Tel: 020 7911 5082
Fax: 020 7911 5079
Email: cavadmin@mwmin.ac.uk
Website: www.wmin.ac.uk/CCCPH

Wolverhampton University
(Complementary Therapies BSc
(Hons))
Contact: T Crossfield
Address: Wulfruna Street,
Wolverhampton, Staffordshire
WV1 1SB
Tel: 01902 321054

ACUPUNCTURE

**Centre for Community Care &
Primary Health, Traditional
Chinese Medicine**
Address: University of
Westminster, 115 New Cavendish
Street, London W1M 8JS
Tel: 020 7911 5000 ext. 3776/+44
Website: www.westminster.ac.uk

**The College of Integrated
Chinese Medicine**
Address: 19 Castle Street,
Reading, Berks RG1 7SB
Tel: 0118 950 8880
Website: www.cicm.org.uk

**The College of Traditional
Acupuncture**
Address: Tao House, Queensway,
Royal Leamington Spa,
Warwickshire CV31 3LZ
Tel: 01926 422121
Website: www.acupuncture-coll.ac.uk

Coventry University (MSc,
PgCert & PgDip)
Contact: Panos Barlas

Address: Priory Street, Coventry,
Warwickshire CV1 5FB
Tel: 024 7683 8980

**The International College of
Oriental Medicine UK**
Address: Green Hedges House,
Green Hedges Avenue, East
Grinstead, West Sussex RH19 1DZ
Tel: 01342 313106
Website: www.orientalmed.ac.uk

**The London College of
Traditional Acupuncture**
Address: HR House, 447 High
Road, Finchley, London N12 0AZ
Tel: 020 8371 0820
Website: www.lcta.com

**The Northern College of
Acupuncture**
Address: 124 Acomb Road, York
YO2 4EY
Tel: 01904 785120/784828
Website: www.chinese-medicine.co.uk

Westminster University (BSc (Hons))
Address: 309 Regent Street,
Westminster, London W1R 8AL
Tel: Cavendish Campus
Admissions – 0207 911 5883

THE ALEXANDER TECHNIQUE

Alexander ReEducation Centre
Address: 10 Langdon Avenue,
Bedgrove Meadows, Aylesbury,
Buckinghamshire HP21 9UX
Tel: 01296 580197

The Alexander Technique School of Cornwall
Address: 40 Gwithian Towans,
Hayle, Cornwall TR27 5BT
Tel: 01739 759526
Fax: 01736 360149
Email: denysstephens@compuserve.com

Brighton Alexander Training Centre
Address: The Rox School of
Dance and Drama, Unit 3, Hove
Business Centre, Fonthill Road,
Hove BN3 6HA
Tel: 01273 501612
Email: jn.nicholls@virgin.net

Bristol Alexander Technique Training School Association
Address: 37 Bellevue Crescent,
Clifton Wood, Bristol, BS8 4TF
Tel: 01179 872989
Fax: 01179 872989
Email: ali.burrows@onet.co.uk

Centre for the Alexander Technique
Address: 46 Stevenage Road,
London SW6 6HA
Tel: 020 7731 6348
Website: www.ribeaux.fsnet.co.uk

Cumbria Alexander Training
Address: Fellside Centre,
Low Fellside, Kendal, Cumbria
LA9 4NH
Tel: 01539 733045
Fax: 01539 724684
Email: jamie@fellside.f9.co.uk

Essex Alexander School
Address: 65 Norfolk Road,
Seven Kings, Ilford, Essex
IG3 8LJ
Tel: 020 8220 1630
Email: ken_thompson@lineone.net
Website: website.lineone.net/
~ken_thompson/index.html

AROMATHERAPY

The Academy of Aromatherapy and Massage
Address: 50 Cow Wynd, Falkirk FK1 1PU
Tel: 01324 612658
Website: www.taams.co.uk

Greenwich University (BSc (Hons))
Address: Wellington Street, Woolwich, London SE18 6PF
Tel: 020 8331 8590

Napier University (BSc modular degree programme)
Contact: Liz Irvine, Programme Leader
Address: 219 Colinton Road, Edinburgh EH14 1DJ
Tel: 01506 42 2880

Oxford Brookes University (BA (Hons))
Address: Gipsy Lane, Headington, Oxford OX3 0BP
Tel: 01865 484848

CHIROPRACTIC

Anglo-European College of Chiropractic (BSc, BSc (Hons), MSc)
Contact: Mrs J Gardiner
Address: 13 Parkwood Road, Bournemouth, Dorset BH5 2DF
Tel: 01202 436200
Email: jgardiner@aecc.ac.uk
Website: www.aecc.ac.uk

Glamorgan University
Address: Chiropractic Field, School of Applied Sciences, Pontypridd, Glamorgan CF37 1DL
Tel: 01443 482287
Fax: 01443 482285
Email: sking@glam.ac.uk
Website: www.glam.ac.uk

Glamorgan University (BSc, BSc (Hons))
Address: Llantwit Road, Treforest, Pontypridd, Rhondda Cynon Taff CF37 1DL
Tel: 01443 480480

McTimoney Chiropractic College Ltd
Address: 14 Park End Street, Oxford OX1 1HH
Tel: 01865 246786

McTimoney Chiropractic College (Distance learning, Access course for those without the necessary science background)
Address: The Clock House, 22–6 Ock Street, Abingdon OX14 5SH
Tel: 01235 523336
Fax: 01235 523576

Email: chiropractic@mctimoney-college.ac.uk
Website: www.mctimoney-college.ac.uk

Portsmouth University (BSc (Hons))
Address: Faculty of Humanities and Social Science, University House, Portsmouth, Hampshire PO1 2UP
Tel: 02392 846010

Surrey University (MSc)
Contact: Dr J Morley, Director of Studies Address: European

Institute of Health & Medical Sciences, Duke of Kent Building, Stag Hill, Guildford, Surrey GU2 5XH
Tel: 01483 879770
Fax: 01483 259395
Email: j.morley@surrey.ac.uk
Website: www.eihms.surrey.ac.uk

Westminster University (BSc (Hons))
Address: 309 Regent Street, Westminster, London W1R 8AL
Tel: Cavendish Campus
Admissions – 020 7911 5883

HERBALISM

College of Integrated Chinese Medicine
Address: 19 Castle Street, Reading, Berks RG1 7SB Tel: 0118 9508 880

College of Phytotherapy
(validated by the University of Wales)
Address: Bucksteep Manor, Bodle Street Green, Nr Hailsham, E Sussex BN27 4RJ
Tel: 01323 834 800
Website:
www.blazeweb.com/phytotherapy/

London College of Traditional Acupuncture & Oriental Medicine
Address: HR House, 447 High Road, Finchley, London N12 0AZ

Tel: 020 8371 0810/0820
Fax: 020 8371 0830

London School of Acupuncture & Traditional Chinese Medicine
Address: University of Westminster, Campus Office, Cavendish Campus, 115 New Cavendish Street, London W1M 8JS
Tel: 020 7911 5000 ext. 3776

Middlesex University
Address: Queens Way, Enfield EN3 4SF Tel: 020 8362 5000
Website: www.mdx.ac.uk/mdx/
academic/course/undergrad/hea/
hmp.htm

The Scottish School of Herbal Medicine (validated by the University of Wales)
Address: Unit 22, Six Harmony Row, Glasgow G51 3BA
Tel: 0141 401 8889
Email: sshm@herbalmedicine.org.uk
Website: www.herbalmedicine.org.uk

Westminster University Address: 115 New Cavendish Street, London W1M 8JS
Tel: 020 7911 5883

Website: www2.wmin.ac.uk/courses/cccph/bschealthsciherbmed.htm

Wolverhampton College (Herbalism and Holistic Health levels 2–3)
Address: Wulfrun Campus, Paget Road, Wolverhampton, Staffordshire WV6 0DU
Tel: 01902 317700

HOMEOPATHY

The British Institute of Homeopathy (Home study and online courses at Diploma level for homeopaths, pharmacists and veterinary surgeons. Also a Postgraduate Course)
Address: The Registrar, Cygnet House, Market Square, Staines, Middlesex TW18 4RH
Tel: 01784 440467
Fax: 01784 449887
E-mail: britinsthom@compuserve.com

British School of Homeopathy
Contact: Administrator
Address: Homelands Cottage, Burrington, Umberleigh, Devon EX37 9JH
Tel: 01769 520462
Email: learnhomeopathy@aol.com

The College of Homeopathy (Licentiate of The College of Homeopathy)

Contact: Admissions Officer
Address: 32 Wellbeck Street, London WIM 7PG
Tel: 020 7487 7487
Fax: 020 7487 4299

The College of Practical Homeopathy (Full- and part-time courses as well as short courses for nurses)
Address: 60 Ballards Lane, Finchley Central, London N3 2BY
Tel: 020 8346 7800
Fax: 020 8343 3376
E-mail: prachome@this.is
Website: http://this.is/homoeopathy

London College of Classical Homeopathy (Licentiate Course in Homeopathy)
Address: LCCH Admissions, Hahnemann House, 32 Welbeck Street, Westminster, London W1M 7PG

Tel: 020 7487 4322
Fax: 020 7487 4299

The Northern College of Homeopathic Medicine
Contact: The Office Manager
Address: First Floor, Swinburne House, Swinburne Street, Gateshead, Tyne & Wear NE8 1AX
Tel: 0191 490 0276

North West College of Homeopathy (Diploma Course in Classical Homeopathy)
Contact: W McTaggart
Address: 23 Wilbraham Road, Fallowfield, Manchester M14 6FG
Tel/Fax: 0161 257 2445

Purton House School of Homeopathy (Diploma in Homeopathy)
Contact: Penley Grange
Address: Marlow Road, Stokenchurch, Buckinghamshire HP14 3UW
Tel: 01753 646625

The School of Homeopathy
Contact: Stuart Gracie
Address: Homeopathic Training, Orchard House, Merthyr Road, Llanfoist, Abergavenny NP7 9LN
Tel: 01873 856872
Fax: 01873 858962

Scottish School of Homeopathy (BSc (Hons))
Contact: Mrs Mary Hood
Address: 21 Abercromby Place, Edinburgh EH3 6QE
Tel: 0131 558 9988

The Yorkshire School of Homeopathy
Contact: John Wise, Registrar
Address: Lansdown, 24 Rosebank, Burley-in-Wharfedale, Ilkley, West Yorkshire LS29 7PQ
Tel/Fax: 01943 862549

HYPNOTHERAPY

Academy of Curative Hypnotherapists Ltd
(Hypnotherapy Foundation Certificate. Also two-year hypnotherapy diploma)
Contact: Simon Kilner
Address: Cheadle Hulme Natural Health Centre, 17 Station Road, Cheadle Hulme, Greater Manchester SK8 5AF
Tel: 0161 485 4009

London College of Clinical Hypnosis (Medical Diploma in Clinical Hypnotherapy)
Contact: Dr R Dupe
Address: 229a Sussex Gardens, Kensington and Chelsea, London W2 2RL
Tel: 020 7706 3360

MASSAGE

Bury College (Sports Massage Diploma)
Address: Market Street, Bury, Manchester BL9 0BG
Tel: 0161 280 8280

Cambridge College of Therapeutic Massage
Address: 5 Dovehouse Close, Fowlmere, Cambs SG8 7SE
Tel: 01763 208388

Clare Maxwell-Hudson School of Massage (Aromatherapy, MLD, Sports Massage)
Address: PO Box 457, London NW2 4BR
Tel: 020 8450 6494
Fax: 020 8208 1639

European Institute of Massage
Address: 27 Martello Park, Seahill, Holywood, Co Down, N. Ireland BT18 0DG
Tel: 01238 425020
Email: jearls@eim.dnet.com

The European School of Healing and Complementary Medicine Ltd (Therapeutic Massage, Lymphatic Drainage)
Address: 34 Downside Road, Sutton, Surrey SM2 5HP
Tel/Fax: 020 8643 1609
Email: 06175.336@compuserve.com

Luton University (Sports Massage and Remedial Therapy BSc (Hons))
Address: Park Square, Luton, Bedfordshire LU1 3JU
Tel: 01582 734111

North Tyneside College (Remedial Massage Diploma)
Address: Embleton Avenue, Wallsend, Tyne and Wear NE28 9NJ
Tel: 0191 229 5000

Revival School of Aromatherapy (Aromatherapy Theory, Massage/Bodywork, Counselling, Client care, Ethics, A&P, EST Practice, Post-grad/Top-up courses)
Address: 120 The Boulevard, Wylde Green, Sutton Coldfield B73 5JG
Tel: 01213 551554
Email: in6075@wiv.ac.uk

Sheffield Centre of Massage Training
Address: 289 Abbydale Road, Sheffield S7 1FJ
Tel: 01142 888317

Thanet College (Sports Massage Certificate)
Address: Ramsgate Road, Broadstairs, Kent CT10 1PN
Tel: 01843 605040

Westminster University (Therapeutic Massage BA (Hons))
Address: 309 Regent Street, Westminster, London W1R 8AL
Tel: 020 7911 5883

NUTRITION

British College of Naturopathy & Osteopathy (BSc (Hons) in Osteopathic Medicine combined with a Naturopathic Diploma, also BSc (Hons) in Naturopathic Medicine (this course is only open to registered medical practitioners, osteopaths, chiropractors and medical herbalists and other practitioners trained in anatomy, physiology, pathology, diagnosis and clinical methods to primary health care levels).
Website: www.bcno.ac.uk/

Glasgow University (Clinical Nutrition MSc)
Address: University Avenue, Glasgow G12 8QQ
Tel: 0141 330 4575

Nottingham University (Clinical Nutrition Certificate/Diploma distance learning)
Contact: Professor I A MacDonald
Address: University Park, Nottingham NG7 2RD
Tel: 0115 970 9475

Queen Margaret University College (Community Nutrition MSc. PgCert. PgDip)
Contact: Jackie Landman
Address: Admissions Office, Clerwood Terrace, Edinburgh EH12 8TS
Tel: 0131 317 3625

South Bank University (Food, Nutrition and Health BSc (Hons))
Address: 103 Borough Road, Southwark, London SE1 0AA
Tel: 020 7815 8158

University of Wales Institute (Applied Human Nutrition BSc (Hons))
Contact: Mrs M Barasi
Address: Student Recruitment & Admissions Office, Western Avenue, Cardiff CF5 2SG
Tel: 029 2041 6878

REFLEXOLOGY

Academy School of Reflexology
Address: 79 Clare Street, Northampton NN1 3JE Tel: 01604 631 806

ARC School of Reflexology
Address: St Pauls House, Edison Road, Bromley, Kent BR2 0EP
Tel: 020 8650 0896

Email: pressure-points@bigfoot.com Website: www.nur.win-uk.net/arc.htm

Caritas School of Reflexology
Address: 24a Chilwell Road, Beeston, Nottingham NG9 1EJ
Tel: 0115 925 8345

Cheltenham School of Reflexology
Address: Lavender Cottage, 5 Church Row, Chedworth, Glos GL54 4AD
Tel: 01285 720131 Email: sarahtromans@lineone.net

Cheryl Butler School of Reflexology
Address: 70 Solway Avenue, Brighton, Sussex BN1 8UJ
Tel: 01273 708307
Fax: 01273 502347
Email: cherylbutler@reflexology.co.uk
Website: www.reflexology.uk.co

Coventry Technical College
(Reflexology Diploma)
Address: Butts, Coventry, Warwickshire CV1 3GD
Tel: 024 7652 6700

Napier University (Part-time BSc modular degree programme)
Contact: Liz Irvine, Programme Leader
Address: 219 Colinton Road, Edinburgh EH14 1DJ
Tel: 01506 42 2880

Oxford School of Reflexology
Address: 45a High Street, Wheatley, Oxon OX33 1XX
Tel: 01865 876 266
Fax: 01865 558 529

Practitioners School of Reflexology
Address: 47 Leyborne Park, Kew, Richmond, Surrey TW9 3HB
Tel/Fax: 020 8948 2380

Rainbow Star School for Reflexologists
Address: Brightlands, North Green Road, Pulham St Mary, Norfolk IP21 4YG
Tel: 01379 608292

Rosalind Oxenford School of Reflexology Address:
Beachwood Cottage, Lansdown, Bath BA1 9DB
Tel: 0117 932 2912
Fax: 0117 932 3137

School of Precision Reflexology
Address: 38 South Street, Exeter EX1 1ED
Tel: 01392 499360

Scottish School of Reflexology
Address: Sheninghurst, 2 Wheatfield Rd, Ayr, Scotland KA7 2XB
Tel/Fax: 01292 287142

SHIATSU

The Bath School of Shiatsu
Contact: Frank Davis
Address: 130 London Road West,
Bath BA1 7DD
Tel: 01225 859209
Email: frankshiatsuyoga@ic24.net

Coventry Technical College
(Shiatsu Intermediate Diploma)
Address: Butts, Coventry,
Warwickshire CV1 3GD
Tel: 024 7652 6700

The Devon School of Shiatsu
Contact: Oliver Cowmeadow
Address: The Coach House,
Buckyette Farm, Littlehempston,
Totnes TQ9 6ND
Tel: 01803 762593
Fax: 01803 762593
Email: devon@devonshiatsu.co.uk
Website: www.devonshiatsu.co.uk

De Montfort University (Shiatsu
Certificate)
Address: School of Art and
Design, Wordsworth Street,
Lincoln, Lincolnshire LN1 3BP
Tel: 01522 512912

The European Shiatsu School
(Bristol)
Contact: Jane Pollard
Address: ESS Bristol,
92 Mina Road, St Werburgh's,
Bristol BS2 9XW
Tel: 0117 955 2117
Fax: 0117 955 2117

Email: jwdpollard@aol.com
Website: www.shiatsu.org.uk

The European Shiatsu School
(Dartford)
Contact: Tony Booker
Address: The Bridge Clinic,
Brent Way, Dartford DA2 6DA
Tel: 01322 279907
Email: tony.booker@virgin.net
Website: www.shiatsu.org.uk

London College of Shiatsu
Contact: Veronica Howard/
Nik Kyriacou
Address: 5–27 Dalling Road,
Ravenscourt Park, London
W6 0JD
Tel: 020 8741 3323
Email:
info@londoncollegeofshiatsu.com
Website:
www.londoncollegeofshiatsu.com

Northern School of Shiatsu
(Shiatsu Diploma)
Contact: Carol Dean
Address: 33 Idsworth Road,
Sheffield, South Yorkshire S5 6UN
Tel: 0114 242 3671

The Shiatsu College (Brighton)
Contact: Briony Young
Address: Brighton Natural
Health Centre, 27 Regents Street,
Brighton BN1 1UL
Tel: 01273 600010
Fax: 01273 600514

Fax: 0131 661 6052
Email: shiatsu@ednet.co.uk

The Shiatsu College (Newcastle upon Tyne)
Contact: Anne Palmer
Address: 39 Manor House Road, Jesmond, Newcastle upon Tyne NE2 2LY

Tel: 0191 281 8201
Fax: 0191 281 8201
Email: ap.shiatsu@dial.pipex.com
Website: www.shiatsucollege.co.uk

The Shiatsu College (Norwich)
Contact: Clifford Andrews
Address: 20a Lower Goat Lane, Norwich NR2 1EL
Tel: 01603 632555
Fax: 01603 663391
Email: admin@shiatsucollege.co.uk
Website: www.shiatsucollege.co.uk

67

LEAD AND PROFESSIONAL BODIES

This section looks at some of the professional (lead) bodies in the UK. Through them, you can access their accredited schools throughout the country.

ACUPUNCTURE

There are five associations representing non-statutory registered health professionals who practise acupuncture. By far the largest of these is the British Acupuncture Council that represents around 2020 acupuncture practitioners. It is associated with the British Acupuncture Accreditation Board which, under an independent chairman, works with the relevant training courses to set out and audit standards of education and training.

British Acadamy of Western Acupuncture
Address: 12 Poulton Green Close, Spital, Wirral, Merseyside L63 9FS
Tel: 0151 3439168/01695 576614

British Acupuncture Council
The BAcC was formed in June 1995 by the unification of five member groups of the Council for Acupuncture (the British Acupuncture Association & Register, The Chung San Acupuncture Society, The International Register of Oriental Medicine, The Register of Traditional Chinese Medicine, and the Traditional Acupuncture Society). The BAcC believes that anyone who wishes to provide acupuncture treatment should undertake an extensive training, regardless of any other qualifications or prior western medical training, and does not endorse short courses.

All practitioner members of the BAcC have undergone a thorough training in traditional acupuncture diagnosis and treatment, comprising a course of study lasting at least two years full time, or the part-time equivalent. Western medical training appropriate to the practice of acupuncture is considered an essential component of such courses, as are both clinical acupuncture training and practical work. Training courses are monitored by the British Acupuncture Accreditation Board (BAAB), an independent body closely allied to BAcC, which was established in 1990 to provide professional accreditation in this field.

Address: British Acupuncture Council
          63 Jeddo Road, London W12 9HQ
Tel: 020 8735 0400
Fax: 020 8735 0404
Email: info@acupuncture.org.uk
Website: www.acupuncture.org.uk

British Medical Acupuncture Society
The British Medical Acupuncture Society (BMAS) represents medically qualified doctors who practise acupuncture alongside conventional medicine. The majority of members are GPs, many of whom offer acupuncture on the NHS.

Address: British Medical Acupuncture Society
          Newton House, Newton Lane, Whitley, Warrington, Cheshire
          WA4 4JA
Tel: 01925 730727
Fax: 01925 730492
Email: bmasadmin@aol.com
Website: www.medical-acupuncture.co.uk

Traditional Acupuncture Society
Address: 1 The Ridgeway, Stratford-upon-Avon CV37 9RD
Tel: 01789 299228

THE ALEXANDER TECHNIQUE

Professional Association of Alexander Teachers
Address: 20 High Street, Norton, Stockton-on-Tees TS20 1DN
Tel: 01642 363542

The Society of Teachers of the Alexander Technique
The Society of Teachers of the Alexander Technique represents about 90 per cent of therapists. They are the core group taking part in wider discussions to create a new general council of teachers of the Alexander Technique.

Address: 129 Camden Mews, London NW1 9AH
Tel: 020 7284 3338
Fax: 020 7482 5435
Email: info@stat.org.uk
Website: www.stat.org.uk/

AROMATHERAPY

There are 12 organisations representing aromatherapists who practise in the UK. Eleven of these are members of an umbrella association, the Aromatherapy Organisations Council (AOC), which provides common codes of ethics and disciplinary procedures and represents the profession in legislative discussions. The AOC is seen as an early precedent for trying to unite professional groups, but there are signs of moves within some of the bodies they represent to establish their own working groups.

Aromatherapy Organisations Council
The AOC is the governing body for aromatherapy and represents 12 professional associations, their 115 or so accredited training establishments and their 6000 therapists. National occupational standards for aromatherapy, developed over a three-year period, were published in June 1998 and agreement has been reached with Middlesex University to develop a BSc Degree in aromatherapy.

Contact: Ms Nina Ashby, Secretary
Address: The AOC
          PO Box 19834, London SE25 6WF
Tel: 020 8251 7912
Fax: 020 8251 7942
Website: www.aromatherapy.uk.com

Federation of Aromatherapists
Address: Stamford House, 2–4 Chiswick High Road, London W4 1TH
Tel: 020 8742 2605

CHIROPRACTIC

British Chiropractic Association
The British Chiropractic Association was established in 1925 and now represents over 800 UK chiropractors. It has strict codes of conduct and ethics. Only chiropractors who have trained for at least four years full time at an accredited college can become members.

Address: British Chiropractic Association
              Blagrave House, 17 Blagrave Street, Reading, Berkshire
              RG1 1QB
Tel: 0118 950 5950
Fax: 0118 958 8946
Email: britchiro@aol.com
Website: www.chiropractic-uk.co.uk

General Chiropractic Council
The General Chiropractic Council (GCC) is a UK-wide statutory body with regulatory powers, established by the Chiropractors Act 1994. Through its Education Committee the GCC sets UK-wide standards of training and competence, ensuring that chiropractors are properly qualified.

Contact: Gregory Price, Executive Director
Address: General Chiropractic Council
              344–354 Gray's Inn Road, London WC1X 8BP
Tel: 020 7713 5155
Fax: 020 7713 5844
Email: enquiries@gcc-uk.org
Website: www.gcc-uk.org

McTimoney Chiropractic Association
The McTimoney Chiropractic Association governs the code of ethics of those practitioners trained at the McTimoney Chiropractic College. It maintains a register of practitioners and issues a directory of McTimoney Chiropractors.

Contact: Mrs Helen Bishop, Administration Manager
Address: McTimoney Chiropractic Association
              21 High Street, Eynsham, Oxon OX8 1HE

Tel: 01865 880974
Fax: 01865 880975
Email   admin@mctimoney-chiropractic.org
Website: www.mctimoney-chiropractic.org

Scottish Chiropractic Association
The Scottish Chiropractic Association was founded in 1979 by seven
chiropractors practising in Scotland. The Association provides the public
with the security of a code of ethics and memorandum and articles that
the membership must abide by. All the members have a certain level of
undergraduate training, with continuing professional development being
encouraged.

Contact: Dr Carla How
Address: Scottish Chiropractic Association
          16 Jenny Moores Road, St Boswells, Roxburghshire, Scotland
          TD6 0AL
Tel: 01835 823645
Fax: 01835 823930
Email: carlahow@scottishborders.co.uk

HERBALISM

Many professional groups are constituent organisations of the new
umbrella body, the European Herbal Practitioners Association
(www.users.globalnet.co.uk/~ehpa/). The Association has declared that it
is actively seeking statutory registration for its members and has been in
discussions with the Department of Health.

British Herbal Medicine Association
The BHMA was founded in 1964 to advance the science and practice of
herbal medicine in the UK and to ensure its continued statutory
recognition at a time when all medicines were becoming subject to
greater regulatory control. Members of the BHMA include companies
involved in the manufacture or supply of herbal medicines or botanical
drugs, herbal practitioners, academics, pharmacists, students of
phytotherapy (the scientific study of plant medicines and their
therapeutic application to relieve illness and promote health) and others.

Address: British Herbal Medicine Association
          Sun House, Church Street, Stroud, Gloucester GL5 1JL
Tel: 01453 751389
Fax: 01453 751402

National Institute of Medical Herbalists
Address: National Institute of Medical Herbalists
          56 Longbrook Street, Exeter, Devon EX4 6AH
Tel: 01392 426022
Fax: 01392 498963
Email: nimh@ukexeter.freeserve.co.uk
Website: www.btinternet.com/~nimh/

Register of Chinese Herbal Medicine
The RCHM is the UK professional body for practitioners of Chinese
herbal medicine (often combined with acupuncture). All members are
bound by strict codes of ethics and practice. Only qualified and
professionally insured practitioners are eligible for membership of the
RCHM. All member practitioners have completed an RCHM-approved
course or equivalent in the UK and/or overseas.

Contact: Mr Melvin Lyons, Development Co-ordinator
Address: Register of Chinese Herbal Medicine
          PO Box 400, Wembley, Middlesex HA9 9NZ
Tel/Fax: 020 7470 8740
Email: herbmed@rchm.co.uk
Website: www.rchm.co.uk

HOMEOPATHY

Two separate groups practise homeopathy: medical homeopaths, who are
medically qualified practitioners regulated by the GMC, and non-
medical homeopaths, who are professionals who use homeopathy only.
There are four main bodies representing the non-medical homeopaths,
the largest of these being the Society of Homeopaths. They have
formally consulted their membership and committed themselves to
pursuing a single register of homeopaths. They have begun to work with
the second largest body, the UK Homeopathic Medical Association
(http://www.homeopathy.org/) and have agreed on national occupational

standards and created a Joint Meeting of Organisations representing professional homeopaths. Although this is evidence of improved co-ordination among professional homeopaths, there has so far been little communication between these groups and the bodies representing medical homeopaths.

British Homeopathic Association
Address: 27a Devonshire Street, London W1N 1RJ
Tel: 020 7935 2163

Society of Homeopaths
The Society of Homeopaths is the largest registering body for professional homeopaths in the UK. Twice a year the Society publishes a Register of Professional Homeopaths who are insured to practise and have completed either a three year full-time or four year part-time course at a recognised college, followed by a minimum of a year's clinical supervision.

Contact: Mrs Mary Clarke, General Secretary
Address: The Society of Homeopaths
                 4 Artisan Road, Northampton NN1 4HU
Tel: 01604 621400
Fax: 01604 622622
Email: societyofhomeopaths@btinternet.com
Website: www.homeopathy.org.uk

HYPNOTHERAPY

There are approximately 17 bodies representing hypnotherapists; five of these are members of the relatively new umbrella body, the UK Confederation of Hypnotherapy Organisations. There are some doctors and dentists who practise hypnotherapy: many are members of the Society of Medical and Dental Hypnosis.

The British Hypnotherapy Association
Address: 67 Upper Berkley Street, London W1H 7DW
Tel: 020 7723 4443

National College of Hypnosis and Psychotherapy
Address: 12 Cross Street, Nelson, Lancashire BB9 7EN
Tel: 01282 699378
Fax: 01282 698633

National School of Hypnosis and Psychotherapy
Address: 28 Finsbury Park Road, London N4 2JX
Tel: 020 7359 6991

MASSAGE

There are approximately nine professional groups representing massage therapists, and two umbrella organisations. The newest of these, the British Association for Massage Therapy, has been most successful at attracting the larger professional bodies and combines the four largest groups. However, it is worth noting that many massage therapists also apply aromatherapy and may therefore be members of aromatherapy organisations or multidisciplinary organisations.

British Federation of Massage Practitioners
Membership of the British Federation of Massage Practitioners (BFMP) has a two-fold benefit. First, your name will be included on the Register for referrals. Secondly, those seeking insurance may be insured through the BFMP.

Contact: Mrs Jolanta Basnyet, Secretary
Address: The British Federation of Massage Practitioners
               78 Meadow Street, Preston, Lancashire PR1 1TS
Tel: 01772 881063
Fax: 01772 881063
Email: Jolanta@Jolanta.co.uk
Website: www.jolanta.co.uk

British Massage Therapy Council
Formed in 1992 by a cross-section of massage therapists from all over the UK, the British Massage Therapy Council (BMTC) has evolved into an umbrella organisation unifying the massage therapy profession, representing a collective voice to the public and the government and setting agreed standards of training supported by a structure of assessment.

Address: The British Massage Therapy Council
           17 Rymers Lane, Oxford OX4 3JU
Tel/Fax: 01865 774123
Email: info@bmtc.co.uk
Website: www.bmtc.co.uk

Society of Massage Therapists
Address: 70 Lochside Road, Denmore Park, Bridge of Don, Aberdeen
           AB23 8QW
Tel: 01224 822596

NUTRITION

Nutritional therapists (non-medical) are currently represented by three main groups, although a new umbrella body, the Nutritional Therapy Council, has recently been set up to focus specifically on education and the development of national occupational standards. The largest of the nutritional therapy groups, the British Association of Nutritional Therapists, sees a chance for the new council to start playing a role in co-ordinating training colleges.

British Association of Nutritional Therapists
Address: British Association of Nutritional Therapists
           BCM BANT, London WC1N 3XX
Tel: 0870 606 1284
Fax: 0870 606 1284

The General Council and Register of Naturopaths
The purpose of the GCRN is to establish and maintain standards of education for practitioners and to provide for the inspection of colleges and courses of naturopathy for the protection and benefit of the public. It encourages the development of naturopathy on the lines of sound knowledge and practice and, to improve the educational standards of members, it also encourages continuing postgraduate education. It provides for and promotes education, investigation and research into the science and art of naturopathy and disseminates the results of such research.

Address: The General Council and Register of Naturopaths
           Goswell House, 2 Goswell Road, Street, Somerset BA16 0JG

Tel: 01458 840072
Fax: 01458 840075
Email: admin@naturopathy.org.uk
Website: http://www.naturopathy.org.uk/

Naturopathic and Osteopathic Association
Address: 6 Netherhall Gardens, London NW3 5RR
Tel: 020 7435 6464

REFLEXOLOGY

There are many groups representing reflexologists, and there have been attempts to achieve consensus among them over recent years, particularly on agreeing national occupational standards for the discipline. The recently launched Reflexology Forum aims to represent every reflexologist in the country.

Association of Reflexologists
The Association is an independent, non-profit-making organisation with a membership of over 5500 reflexologists. Although not affiliated to any particular school, the Association accredits practitioner courses when they meet the high standards set and maintained by the Association's Schools Council. A list of accredited practitioner courses, conducted at over 95 centres in the UK and Eire, is published and updated four times a year.

Address: Association of Reflexologists
          27 Old Gloucester Street, London WC1N 3XX
Tel: 0870 567 3320
Email: aor@reflexology.org
Website: www.reflexology.org/aor/

British Reflexology Association
Address: Monks Orchard, Whitbourne, Worcester WR6 5RB
Tel: 01886 821207
Fax: 01886 822017

International Federation of Reflexologists
The IFR was formed in the 1980s. As well as keeping a register of professional therapists, the IFR has a list of accredited schools which all teach to a centrally agreed syllabus.

Address: International Federation of Reflexologists
Croydon, Surrey CR0 1EF
Tel: 020 8667 9458
Fax: 020 8649 9291
Email: ifr44@aol.com
Website: www.reflexology-ifr.com

SHIATSU

Over the past two years two new Shiatsu bodies have been created, resulting in five bodies overall. The Shiatsu Society, the oldest and largest, supports the idea of statutory regulation, while the other Shiatsu bodies believe Shiatsu should remain voluntarily regulated.

Shiatsu Society (UK) Ltd
The Shiatsu Society (UK) has become a recognised and respected independent professional association. The Society took on the self-regulating role of maintaining professional standards of practice and training and has now become the main professional association for practitioners, teachers and training establishments within the UK.

Contact: Samantha Chadband, Administrator
Address: The Shiatsu Society (UK)
Eastlands Court, St Peters Road, Rugby, Warwickshire CV21 3QP
Tel: 01788 555051
Fax: 01788 555052
Email: admin@shiatsu.org
Website: www.shiatsu.org

UMBRELLA ORGANISATIONS

British Complementary Medicine Association
The BCMA is the major complementary medicine, multi-therapy umbrella body in the UK, representing some 45 single therapy organisations (some of which are in themselves umbrella bodies but for a single therapy) and some 18 independent schools. Through this structure it speaks for over 20,000 practitioners of 11 different therapies. The BCMA operates a system of voluntary self-regulation with a code of conduct and a complaint

investigation and disciplinary procedure, which are mandatory for all members and their practitioners. All applicants for membership undergo an investigation to ensure they have a satisfactory standard of education and training as part of their entry requirements. A minimum level of medical negligence and public liability insurance is also a requirement. It is also moving towards a requirement for continuing professional development for membership and maintains a practitioner register for referrals of suitably qualified practitioners to the public. It is encouraging all its members i) to become involved in the development of national occupational standards through Healthcare UK and the Qualifications and Curriculum Authority as part of its commitment to ongoing standard-raising, and ii) to seek voluntary statutory self-regulation as is available under the recent Health Act.

Address: The British Complementary Medicine Association
           Kensington House, 33 Imperial Square, Cheltenham
           GL50 1QZ
Tel: 01242 519911
Fax: 01242 227765
Email: info@bcma.co.uk
Website: www.bcma.co.uk

Complementary Medicine Association
Address: The Meridian, 142a Greenwich High Road, London SE10 8NN
Tel: 020 8305 9571

Council for Complementary and Alternative Medicine
Address: Suite D, Park House, 206–208 Latimer Road, London W10 6RE
Tel: 020 8968 3862

The Foundation for Integrated Medicine
The Foundation was formed at the personal initiative of HRH The Prince of Wales, who is now the President. Its aim is to promote the integrated delivery of safe, effective and efficient forms of healthcare, including orthodox and complementary medicine, through greater collaboration between all forms of healthcare.

Address: International House, 59 Compton Road, London N1 2YT
Tel: 020 7688 1881
Fax: 020 7688 1882
Email: enquiries@fimed.org
Website: www.fimed.org

FURTHER RESOURCES

Getting into Self-Employment, Joanna Grigg, Trotman

How to Work from Home, Ian Phillipson, How To Books

How to Start a Business from Home, Graham Jones, How To Books

Students' Money Matters, Gwenda Thomas, Trotman

University Scholarships & Awards, Brian Heap, Trotman

Amazon.co.uk (www.amazon.co.uk) offers a comprehensive list of books on complementary therapies and self-employment.

The Internet Health Library (www.internethealthlibrary.com) is the leading Internet health resource focusing on complementary medicine and natural healthcare, and it is the official health information provider for the British Complementary Medicine Association.

GENERAL BOOKS ON COMPLEMENTARY THERAPIES

Aromatherapy for Health Professionals, S Price, L Price and D Penoel, Churchill Livingstone

Basics of Acupuncture, G Stux and B Pomeranz, Springer-Verlag

Body Massage: Therapy basics, M Rosser, Hodder & Stoughton Educational

Chiropractic, W H Koch, Bayeux Arts

The Complete Homeopathy Handbook: A guide to everyday health care, M Castro, St Martin's Press

The Complete Illustrated Guide to the Alexander Technique: A practical program for health, poise, and fitness, Glynn MacDonald and Glenn MacDonald, Element

Hypnosis for Change, J Hadley & C Staudacher, New Harbinger Publications

Living Wisdom: Herbalism, F J Lipp, Pan

The Optimum Nutrition Bible, P Holford, Piatkus Books

The Reflexology Handbook, L Norman and T Coran, Piatkus Books

Shiatsu: The complete guide, C Jarmey, HarperCollins

Careers-Portal
the Online Careers Service

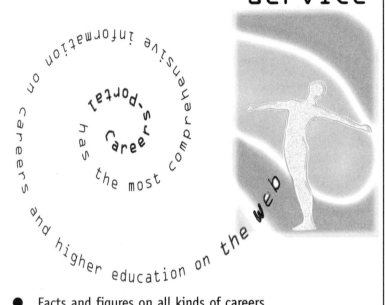

Careers-Portal has the most comprehensive information on careers and higher education on the web

- Facts and figures on all kinds of careers
- HE: Uncovered
- Over 2000 links to universities, job & careers sites
- Art & Design – the guide to winning the HE place you want
- £3000 up for grabs in our 'Win Your Rent' competition
- And lots more...

So come online and see for yourself the advertising potential!

www.careers-portal.co.uk

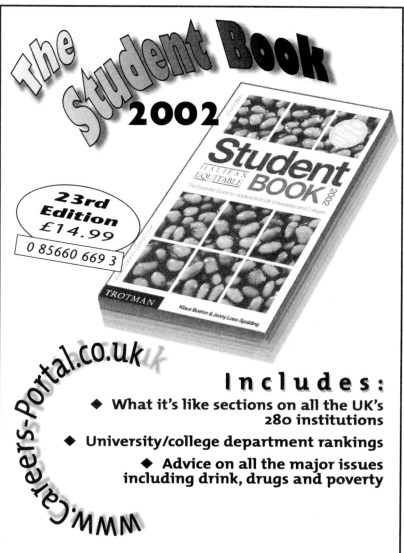

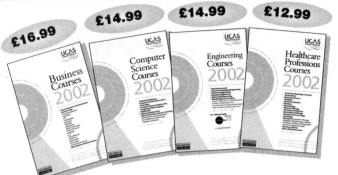
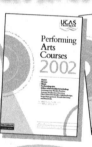
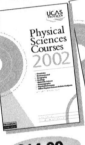
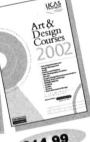